Neurological Examination of the Child with Minor Neurological Dysfunction

T0260663

Neurological Examination of the Child with Minor Neurological Dysfunction

THIRD EDITION

Mijna Hadders-Algra

Professor of Developmental Neurology,
Department of Paediatrics – Developmental Neurology,
University Medical Center Groningen,
Groningen, the Netherlands

2010
Mac Keith Press

© 2010 The Author.

Editor: Hilary M. Hart
Managing Director, Mac Keith Press: Caroline Black
Production Manager: Udoka Ohuonu
Project Manager: Annalisa Welch
Indexer: Laurence Errington

First published in this edition 2010 by
Mac Keith Press, 2nd Floor, Rankin Building, 139-143 Bermondsey Street, London SE1 3UW, UK

Reprinted 2013, 2015, 2016, 2018, 2019, 2022

British Library Cataloguing-in-Publication data
A catalogue record of this book is available from the British Library

ISBN: 978–1–898683–98–8

Typeset by Keystroke Typesetting and Graphic Design Ltd, Tettenhall, Wolverhampton

Print managed by Jellyfish Solutions

Contents

Foreword

I write this foreword with great pleasure. For two reasons. In the first place it gives me the opportunity to express my gratitude and my admiration for the splendid way in which Professor Hadders-Algra has revised and updated this book. The book has practically been rewritten. This became desirable as the first edition was published in 1970 and its second – and until now last – edition dates from 1979. Although the technique of the examination remained the same over the years far more is now known about the details, meaning, and background of minor neurological dysfunction. Theoretical considerations have changed and ideas about the cause and origin of many a minor sign have changed with them. So the book urgently required an update. And I am happy to say that Professor Hadders-Algra has undertaken this task in her well-known clear and reliable way.

The second reason why I am delighted to be writing this foreword is that it gives me the opportunity to say something about the history of the book. The examination presented here is part of developmental neurology and developmental neurology is closely connected with the name of Heinz Prechtl. In the 1950s he presented his concept that instead of being a miniature adult the child of any age has his own, age-appropriate brain with its own age-appropriate function. Consequently the child's nervous system requires a developmental approach, that is to say, the developing brain requires age-adapted examination techniques, based on a close observation of the child's sensorimotor behaviour.

The need for a developmental approach had of course long been appreciated by paediatricians, but it had not yet reached neurological practice. Moreover, the changing characteristics of the developing normal brain were largely unknown at the time. It stands to reason that this concept had a considerable effect on the early detection of brain diseases in infancy and childhood, and also on the appraisal of mild deviations of brain function. In Groningen we carried out neurological examinations of year cohorts of newborn infants and did follow-up studies of infants who were considered to be at risk of neurological dysfunction. These studies enabled us to formulate age-appropriate and standardized examination techniques for newborn infants and older children.

I had the honour of being Professor Prechtl's co-worker in the latter half of the last century and I helped him in developing his concept for older infants and preschool and school-age children. Texts on neurological development in infancy and on an age-adapted technique for examination of (pre-)school children were the result.

The first edition of the present book appeared in 1970 with Professor Prechtl as co-author. In 1979 the book underwent its first revision and expansion. In those years behavioural and learning problems in otherwise normal children were considered to be based on brain abnormalities – that is to say, on neurological dysfunctions that might be mild or even hardly detectable. During the last quarter of the twentieth century psychological and psychiatric concepts came (again) to the fore. Perhaps this was a reason for a decreasing interest in minor neurological signs of dysfunction. However, gradually the insight grew that both psychiatric and somatic (including genetic) causes might play a role in behavioural and learning problems in children. So there is, once more, an increasing demand for a proper and age-adequate neurological appraisal of a child's functioning. And a new edition of 'my manual' seemed desirable.

Professor Hadders-Algra, who joined us in the early 1980s, is an expert on the analysis of the variety of signs that might be found in children. She has managed to pinpoint the signs with the greatest clinical significance and also those signs of less significance. The results of much of her work can be found in the present edition of this book. Moreover she has been able to condense and summarize in a very readable way the many publications of the last 50 years or so on the significance of mild signs of neurological dysfunction and their possible relationship with the problems of children with neurodevelopmental disorders. As a result the present book has more to offer than a mere examination technique.

Reading the new edition I could sometimes hardly recognize it; I consider this to be a compliment. This compliment is a proper end to a foreword to a magnificent rewrite of a book that lies close to my heart.

Bert C L Touwen
Emeritus Professor of Developmental Neurology
Groningen University, The Netherlands

Foreword

Clinicians are often asked to see children whose motor development – although not associated with abnormalities of formal neurological examination – is clearly at the 'end of the bell curve' and causing concern to parents, and sometimes very real functional problems, frustration and unhappiness to the child. This book will be of great assistance to therapists and developmental paediatricians seeing these children.

Faced with clinical findings of uncertain significance the clinician is wise to counsel 'watching and waiting'. The problem is that we are generally better at the waiting than the watching, and thus have not been learning as well as we should have been about 'soft' neurological signs and what we can infer from them, over the many years since our attention was first drawn to them.

Mijna Hadders-Algra has been watching: carefully and over many years. The honesty and objectivity with which she has approached this important topic is exemplary. When she realized that earlier data actually don't fully support previous conclusions she has said so. She has not been afraid to revise previous work and in this, the third edition of the book, the examination schema has been simplified and improved in light of field testing. She has also recognized the limited inter-observer reliability of previous forms of the examination, identified a major cause in inconsistent technique and, in the major change in this edition, has set about improving this through inclusion of still and video footage. Her attention to detail and determination to bring one area of clinical enquiry to some clear conclusions are exemplary.

A researcher of her integrity is not blind to remaining questions. In this, as in other areas very familiar to all clinicians involved in child development, the limitations of arbitrary thresholds of 'caseness' for a continuously distributed ability are well-known. We all recognize the inadequacies of binary labels such as dyspraxia ('Has my child got it? Yes or no?') concepts. The limited correlation between findings of signs of minimal brain dysfunction and magnetic resonance imaging findings underline this, and are fully discussed, but unless and until clinicians' assessment is supplanted by a 'scan 'em all' mentality, the many years of careful work this book represents will be valued by all working in the field.

Rob J Forsyth
Consultant and Senior Lecturer in Child Neurology
Newcastle General Hospital and Newcastle University
Newcastle upon Tyne, UK

Acknowledgements

First and foremost I thank Professor Bert Touwen who taught me the principles of developmental neurology and the basics of the neurological examination of children. He always stressed the need for a standardized, age-specific, and comprehensive neurological assessment in children with motor, learning, and behavioural disorders. In addition he underlined that simple one-to-one relationships do not exist in the field of neurobehavioural and neurocognitive associations. I feel privileged that I was allowed to rewrite the manual that he developed in the 1970s and I thank him for his encouragement and warm support during the process of rewriting.

Karel Maathuis, MD, PhD and Jessika van Hoorn, MD, are kindly acknowledged for their critical comments on earlier drafts of the chapters. Thank you to Loes de Weerd for secretarial assistance. Michiel Schier, Msc, was a great help in the preparation of the figures and the videos for the manual. He also developed the electronic version of the assessment form on the DVD.

Last but not least, I thank the children who volunteered for the pictures and who allowed us to use the videos of their performance. The parents of the children whose pictures or videos are included in the manual and the children older than 9 years whose videos were used provided written permission for the use of their photographs and videos.

Media

Assessment forms and videos, illustrating typical and atypical performance, accompany the book and are FREE to download with every book purchase.

Contact **admin@mackeith.co.uk** for free access if you have purchased the book from another book seller

Chapter 1
Introduction

The presentation of a specific and rather extensive neurological examination of children aimed at the detection of minor deviations in their neurological functions requires some justification. Why are the usual neurological techniques employed by many neuropaediatricians and neurologists insufficient? This question can be divided into two: why a specific examination for children and why an examination for minor deviations?

The answer to the first question is that a child's nervous system is qualitatively different from that of an adult. It is a rapidly developing nervous system, whereas the adult's has reached a relatively stable phase of development. The most dramatic neuro-developmental changes occur during prenatal life and the first postnatal years. However, many changes also take place even after 2 years of age (Figure 1.1). For instance, dendritic growth of cortical neurons is first completed around the age of 5 (Koenderink and Uylings, 1995). Yet, the most prominent changes in the brain after preschool age consist of complex and abundant synaptic reorganization, brought about by synapse formation, synapse elimination, and myelination (De Graaf-Peters and Hadders-Algra, 2006). These developmental changes are associated with a steady growth of the brain during childhood and adolescence. The growth is the net result of thinning of cortical grey matter and thickening of cortical white matter (Sowell et al, 2004; Wilke et al, 2007). The thinning of cortical grey matter is a global process with regional differences. The most prominent thinning occurs in the occipital and right frontal areas, whereas in the anterior and posterior perisylvian regions, i.e. in Broca's and Wernicke's areas, grey matter changes consist of thickening not thinnning (Sowell et al, 2004). White matter changes in school-age children including adolescents occur especially in prefrontal regions, in the internal capsule as well as in basal ganglia and thalamic pathways, the ventral visual pathways, and the corpus callosum (Barnea-Goraly et al, 2005).

The continuous changes in the developing brain have consequences for the neurological examination, for both the technique and the interpretation of findings. This implies that

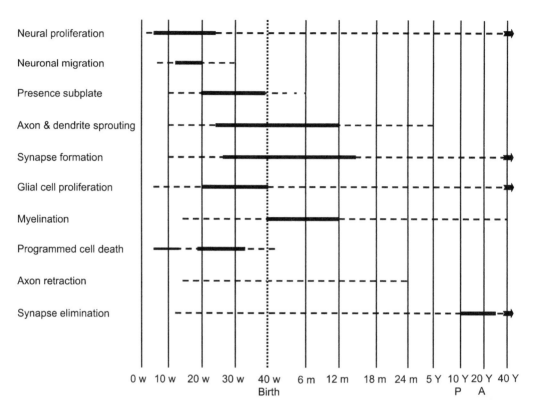

Figure 1.1 Summary of timing of neurobiological processes in the telencephalon during human ontogeny. The subplate is a functionally important transient structure in the telencephalon. A broken line means that the process is active, a bold line indicates that the process is very active. Note that the time axis at the bottom of the figure is an arbitrary one. A, onset of adulthood; m, postnatal months; P, onset of puberty;. w, weeks; Y, years. Adapted from de Graaf-Peters and Hadders–Algra, 2006.

the examiner must be familiar with the natural history of the neurological repertoire, because some neurological phenomena will merely change with age (e.g. diadochokinesis), whereas others disappear altogether (e.g. many associated movements). Moreover, there are several neurological signs that are specific to childhood. For example choreiform dyskinesia, if present, is usually more prominent during childhood than in adulthood, and minor deviations of gait can be observed more easily during childhood than at a later age when walking is fully differentiated. It is clear, therefore, that an examination technique based on adult neurological functions is inappropriate for use with children because the examiner cannot evaluate the specific properties of the developing nervous system. The method used must be a developmental neurological examination.

The answer to the second question (why an examination for minor deviations?) is related to the indications for neurological examination. Generally speaking, there are three main indications for the neurological examination of children, with particular emphasis on minor deviations.

(1) There is the suspicion of a neurological disease in its initial stage, on the basis of the history of the child's complaints (e.g. headaches and vomiting, or slow deterioration of cognitive and/or motor abilities) or on the basis of family history (e.g. tuberous sclerosis or muscle disease).

(2) There are children with an obvious neurological disorder, such as some form of cerebral palsy, for whom it is important to discover all those facets of their neurological condition that are significant in deciding on treatment. For example, a child with overt unilateral spastic cerebral palsy may be found to have minor coordination difficulties in the least affected hand that require treatment. In both instances the examination technique must be refined enough to enable the examiner to detect slight neurological dysfunction.

(3) The neurological examination is a valuable tool in the assessment of children with learning, behavioural and coordination problems, such as attention-deficit–hyperactivity disorder (ADHD), autistism-spectrum disorder (ASD) and developmental coordination disorder (DCD; American Psychiatric Association, 2000).

It is this third category of children with whom this book is mainly concerned. The purpose is to assist the examiner who is asked about the possibility of neurological dysfunction as a neurobiological base for the aberrant behaviour (see Chapters 2 and 10). The neurological dysfunction, if present, will be minor, so the examination must be detailed and comprehensive in order to scrutinize a large variety of neural mechanisms.

It is essential to have a clear idea of what a neurological examination will reveal. Learning, behavioural and coordination problems are only part of complex patterns of behaviour, defined as a whole set of actions carried out by the child with the purpose of changing his environment, or himself in relation to that environment. Of course, complex behaviour is mediated by the nervous system, but the neurological examination, which by its very nature must be limited, can assess only the part of this behaviour that falls within the scope of the examination itself (e.g. sensorimotor function, posture and motility, reactions and responses). The absence of minor neurological signs is not proof of the perfect integrity of the brain, nor does their presence automatically imply a causal relationship with the manifested behaviour. Although this may be so in some cases – for example clumsy movement in a child with slight coordination deficits or choreiform dyskinesia – it is certainly not so in all cases. This point is discussed further in Chapter 2; here it will suffice to say that a child with behavioural and learning difficulties should be assessed neurologically because the brain is involved in generating his behaviour and the neurological assessment enables the examiner to evaluate at least part of the integrity of the brain. The assessment may not result in a specific diagnosis of the cause of the behavioural disorder but it must still be considered an important part of the diagnostic process.

Obviously the neurological examination should detect dysfunctions or substantiate their absence, but it should also differentiate these impairments from deviations that stem from a lag in the speed of maturation of the brain (i.e. signs of developmental delay). The aim of a refined and age-appropriate examination technique is to differentiate these cases. It is important, too, to emphasize the difference between a neurological examination and a developmental assessment. The latter is mainly concerned with correct performances in accordance with the developmental timetables for any particular behaviour (assessment of *what* the child is able to achieve). The neurological examination, in contrast, is concerned with the way in which the child performs the task, the developmental changes in the performance being taken into account (assessment of *how* the child accomplishes the task; see also Touwen, 1981).

The minimum age for the assessment described in this book is 4 years. Some test items can be assessed at a younger age (e.g. muscle tone, tendon reflexes or the mouth-opening and finger-spreading phenomenon), whereas a few (e.g. the finger opposition test) can only be performed from 5 years onwards. No upper age limit for the examination exists, implying that the assessment is also applicable in adolescents and adults. The assessment is part of the methodological arsenal of the physician working in the field of neuropaediatrics, developmental paediatrics, child and adolescent psychiatry and paediatric rehabilitation. As it concerns the most complex system of the organism, it is not surprising that it involves equally complex methods of examination; these may appear difficult and time consuming, requiring special skills and knowledge. It is impossible, however, to design a series of 'crucial' neurological tests that will indicate whether the brain is functioning typically or atypically. A plea for a short form of neurological screening for this purpose, although understandable, ignores the essential properties of the central nervous system. A test of one single part of the neurological repertoire, for example walking, may give information about that particular function but it will not evaluate the neurological mechanisms on which the function is based, and such evaluation is necessary in the case of inadequate performance. Moreover, the examination of a single aspect of the nervous system – coordination for example – does not give sufficient information about other aspects such as muscle power or reflexes.

It is self-evident that functions such as hearing, speech, and vision must also be assessed carefully at a level of speciality that falls outside the scope of this book. These evaluations should be done separately from the neurological assessment as the combination of assessments would take too much time and would be too fatiguing for the child, giving unreliable results. This book deals only with routine neurological assessment and so it does not cover the assessment of these other functions. For the same reason, other techniques by which the child's brain may be assessed, such as magnetic resonance imaging or electroencephalographic examination, will not be discussed.

The assessment of minor neurological dysfunction (MND) is a criterion-referenced assessment. This means that criteria have been defined for typical and atypical performance. The criteria provided in the book are based on the experience of Bert Touwen and Mijna Hadders-Algra, gathered over a few decades, in the assessment of MND in children and adolescents. The criteria for the items that show little or no developmental change are straightforward: typical behaviour is characterized by the absence of dysfunction, for example the absence of stereotyped posture and motility, the absence of deviancies in muscle tone or reflexes, the absence of dyskinesias, the absence of sensory dysfunction, and of cranial nerve dysfunction. The definition of criteria for typical behaviour in those tests where performance is largely age dependent, such as diadochokinesis or the finger opposition test, is less easy. Performance on these tests is not only affected by the integrity of the brain but also by experience. The latter implies that what is typical for a certain population may be atypical for another population, i.e. a population living in a different area or living in a different time period. The question of whether criteria for typical performance on a neurological test should be adapted to the population or not, has no simple answer. This may be illustrated by the following observation. Over the years we stuck to the 'Groningen norms'; this allowed us to observe that in the 1980s about 10% of children showed a performance on diadochokinesis that was inappropriate for age, whereas more recently this figure has risen to over 50%. At the same time the prevalence of choreiform dyskinesia changed from 13% to 8%. This suggests that neurological conditions in children in the Northern parts of the Netherlands have changed over the years, a change which most likely has a multifactorial origin (Hadders-Algra, 2007). The following factors may play a role:

- increasing maternal age at birth in association with assisted reproductive techniques (Middelburg et al, 2008);
- more surviving very preterm infants (Allen, 2008);
- changes in nutrition such as an increased consumption of pre-prepared food (Bouwstra et al, 2006);
- changes in infant care habits, such as little exposure to the prone position and high exposure to the supine position and sitting semi-reclined in portable infant seats (Monson et al, 2003);
- changes in daily life activities at school age: less outdoor fantasy play and more time spent watching TV and playing computer games (Li et al, 2008).

The uncertainty about the origin of the changes in neurological performance made us decide to stick to the previously defined criteria for typical performance on the individual tests. The criteria are described for each test and illustrated by video examples on the accompanying DVD.

Chapters 4 to 9 deal with the actual assessment procedures. For each item the course of actions is described. This is followed by information on the effect of age on assessment and performance, and details of scoring. This is concluded with an account of the significance of the findings. It should be realized that not all reported significance has a solid scientific foundation. Where possible, details of studies supporting the evidence on the underlying neural substrate of specific findings are given. However, part of the description of the significance of findings is based only on general clinical experience in neurology.

Finally, writing about individuals who may be male or female gives an author an awkward choice of consistent referral to both genders by using expressions such as he/she or the selection of one of the two genders. The latter results in a text which is easier to read, but this option has the disadvantage that an impression of 'neglect' of the other gender occurs. I opted for the single-gender option to facilitate readability, and choose the female gender when referring to the examiner and the male gender when referring to the child. However, I would like to stress my gender-neutral intentions.

Chapter 2
Assessment of minor neurological dysfunction

History: minimal brain dysfunction and minor neurological dysfunction
Interest in the neurological condition of children with learning and behavioural disorders emerged in the first half of the twentieth century. In the 1920s the idea that specific types of behaviour might be regarded as expressions of injury to the child's brain was inspired by the finding that children who recovered from encephalitis developed hyperactivity, antisocial behaviour, and emotional instability (Kessler, 1980). Next, the view that specific behaviour, in particular hyperkinesis, was related to brain injury was strongly promoted by Strauss and Lehtinen (1947) who claimed that hyperactivity, impulsivity, and distractability in children with learning disability were indicators of brain damage. Another element was brought into the discussion by Pasamanick and colleagues, who suggested that learning and behavioural problems were associated with brain dysfunction induced by prenatal and perinatal adversities in a similar way to the prenatal and perinatal origin of most cases of cerebral palsy (the concept of 'continuum of reproductive casualty'; Pasamanick et al, 1956; Kawi and Pasamanick, 1958).

At that time the neurological examination offered one of the best ways to assess the integrity of the child's brain. It was obvious that most children with learning and behavioural disorders did not exhibit frank neurological pathology. Focus shifted to the significance of minor neurological dysfunction (MND). Various assessment techniques were developed, such as the PANESS (Physical And Neurological Examination for Soft Signs; Close, 1973; Denckla, 1985) and the examination of minor neurological dysfunction (the Groningen Assessment; Touwen and Prechtl, 1970; Touwen, 1979).

In the 1960s and 1970s the issue of minimal brain damage or minimal brain dysfunction was discussed (see Kalverboer et al, 1978; Rie and Rie, 1980; Nichols and Chen, 1981). But already in 1962, an international study group concluded that the minimal brain dysfunction concept should be discarded, as the label referred to a very heterogeneous group of children (Bax and Mac Keith, 1963). Gradually, children previously diagnosed as having minimal brain dysfunction obtained more specific diagnoses, such as attention-deficit–hyperactivity disorder (ADHD), pervasive developmental disorder not otherwise specified (PDD–NOS), developmental coordination disorder (DCD) or reading disorder. The application of specific diagnoses was facilitated by the *Diagnostic and Statistical Manual of Mental Disorders* (current edition DSM–IV; American Psychiatric Association 2000).

Concurrent with the discussion about the concept of minimal brain dysfunction the significance of MND was debated. The debate is illustrated by the many terms used for MND, such as 'equivocal signs' (Kennard, 1960), 'soft signs' (Hertzig, 1981), 'nonfocal neurological signs' (Hertzig, 1987) and 'subtle signs' (Denckla, 1985). The following two types of signs were distinguished:

(1) mild forms of 'hard' neurological signs, such as mild hypertonia, reflex asymmetries or choreiform dyskinesia;
(2) developmental signs, such as an age-inappropriate performance of diadochokinesis or the finger opposition test or the presence of an excessive amount of associated movements (Tupper 1987).

The significance of both types of signs was controversial and often regarded as not helpful, as they frequently reflected transient findings that disappeared with age. Moreover their aetiology was considered highly speculative (Schmitt, 1975). Yet, many studies indicated that groups of children with psychiatric disorders, in particular with hyperactivity and attention disorder, and with specific learning difficulties more often exhibited signs of MND than typically developing comparison groups (e.g. Lucas et al, 1965; Stine et al, 1975; Denckla and Rudel, 1978; Nichols and Che, 1981; Hadders-Algra et al, 1988a). Other studies demonstrated relationships between prenatal and perinatal adversities, in particular preterm birth and intrauterine growth retardation, and the development of MND (Nichols and Chen 1981; Hadders-Algra et al, 1988b, 1988c; Largo et al, 1989). However, the studies also indicated that signs of MND are highly prevalent in typically developing children (Nichols and Chen 1981; Hadders-Algra et al 1988b). The general conclusion was that relationships between MND and (1) prenatal and perinatal risk factors and (2) learning and behavioural disorders were statistically significant but clinically irrelevant (e.g. Capute et al, 1981; Berninger and Colwell, 1985).

Meanwhile, a series of studies by Rutter and colleagues had demonstrated that children with known pathology of the brain, such as children with cerebral palsy or epilepsy, or children with severe head injuries, had substantially higher rates of cognitive and behavioural problems than typically developing peers (Rutter et al, 1970, 1980; Brown et al, 1981; Chadwick et al, 1981). Rutter (1982) concluded that mild or subclinical forms of damage to the developing brain may result in cognitive and behavioural dysfunction. He also argued that the risk of behavioural problems after a lesion of the brain is lower than the risk of cognitive disorders as environmental factors play a larger role in the former than in the latter. Finally, he stated that the relation between mild brain damage and cognitive and behavioural problems is unspecific, i.e. a lesion of the brain at an early age does not give rise to a specific type of behavioural disorder or specific types of cognitive dysfunction. If cognition is affected the result is a global decrease in cognitive ability.

Current application of the assessment of MND

More recently novel imaging techniques, such as functional magnetic resonance imaging (MRI), volumetric MRI and diffusion tensor imaging, allow for a relatively precise investigation of the child's brain. The application of the novel imaging techniques has increased our understanding of the neurobiological substrate of specific developmental disorders. The imaging data underlined the clinical notion that developmental disorders, such as ADHD and dyslexia, are not homogeneous entities, but consist of a group of disorders (Pernet et al, 2009; Steinhausen, 2009). For instance children with ADHD may show primarily hyperactive–impulsive behaviour; primarily inattention problems; or a combination of these two problems. The imaging studies also indicated the presence of subtypes of ADHD, e.g. ADHD associated with dysfunction of the prefrontal cortex and basal ganglia and ADHD with cerebellar dysfunction (Krain and Castellanos, 2006). Yet, it is still unknown whether and how the clinical subtypes of ADHD are related to the subtypes found on imaging.

Gradually it also became clear that children with a developmental diagnosis, such as ADHD, often have additional diagnoses (Angold et al, 1999; De Jong et al, 2009). For instance, ADHD may be associated with oppositional defiant disorder, depression, anxiety, or DCD (Gillberg and Kadesjö, 2003; Elia et al, 2008). Interestingly, Batstra et al (2006) demonstrated that the presence of multiple psychiatric diagnoses was more strongly linked with prenatal and perinatal adversities than the presence of a single psychiatric diagnosis. This corresponds to the finding of Sprich-Buckminster et al (1993) that ADHD as a single diagnosis in general has a genetic origin, whereas ADHD that is complicated by psychiatric comorbidity more often can be attributed to adverse conditions during fetal and neonatal life.

The above illustrates that the idea that the brain of children with developmental disorders functions in an atypical way is no longer controversial. However, in individual children the aetiology and pathogenesis of atypical function is usually far from clear. For clinicians, the assessment of MND may offer a tool to document the neurological integrity of the child's brain. The neurological findings may assist the understanding of aetiology and facilitate tailor-made guidance for the child. Currently, the most commonly used methods to assess MND are the Zürich Neuromotor Assessment, the Neurological Examination for Subtle Signs and the examination of minor neurological dysfunction (the Groningen Assessment) developed in Groningen. The methods differ in particular with respect to the degree in which they rely on developmental signs.

The Zürich Neuromotor Assessment
The Zürich Neuromotor Assessment (ZNA; Largo et al, 2001a, 2001b; Schmidhauser et al, 2006; Rousson et al, 2008) is restricted to the assessment of developmental signs. The test consists of a timed assessment of specific motor tasks, such as repetitive movements of the fingers, alternating movements, including diadochokinesis, side-to-side jumping and walking on heels. In addition to recording the duration of performance the degree of associated movements is also assessed. A major advantage of the test is that the main parameter 'time in seconds' can be assessed easily and reliably (Rousson et al, 2008). Another advantage is that the test evaluates relatively complex functions mediated by complex neural mechanisms. This increases the likelihood of an association between adverse test results and developmental disorders (Schmidhauser et al, 2006; Freitag et al, 2007). The disadvantage of the ZNA is that the outcome parameters only provide limited, i.e. unspecific, insight into the function of the child's brain. It is important to appreciate that the ZNA differs from assessments aiming to test the child's motor abilities, such as the Movement Assessment Battery for Children (Movement ABC; Henderson and Sugden, 2007) or the Bruininks–Oseretsky Test of Motor Proficiency (Bruininks, 1978). The latter tests consist of a quantitative evaluation of complex meaningful motor activities, such as putting coins in a box or cutting the picture of an elephant out of a piece of paper, whereas the ZNA consists of a quantitative evaluation of 'isolated' complex motor tasks, such as diadochokinesis.

The Neurological Examination for Subtle Signs
The Neurological Examination for Subtle Signs (NESS; Denckla, 1985) is the revised version of the Physical And Neurological Examination for Soft Signs (PANESS; Close, 1973). It consists of items testing timed motor performance and associated movements like the ZNA, but it also includes items on hand, foot and eye preference, sensory functions (graphaesthesia and stereognosis) and one item on dyskinesia. This means that the NESS combines the quantitative approach of the ZNA with a qualitative evaluation. Reliability studies indicated that the test–retest reliability of the PANESS at item level was moderate to poor, but satisfactory for overall outcome (Werry and Aman, 1976; Holder et al, 1982). Reliability of the NESS has been determined by Vitiello et al (1989). Interrater agreement for the timed items and some of the qualitative items was satisfactory, but poor for the items dealing with associated movements and smoothness. Test–retest agreement after an interval of 2 weeks was poor. Limited information is available on the validity of the PANESS and NESS. It has been reported that PANESS scores for children with ADHD, high-functioning autism, and Aspergers syndrome were higher than that of typically developing comparison children (Denckla and Rudel, 1978; Jansiewicz et al, 2006).

Examination of minor neurological dysfunction (the Groningen Assessment)
This book describes the neurological assessment developed in Groningen by Touwen and Prechtl (Touwen and Prechtl, 1970; Touwen 1979). The assessment includes traditional neurological items, such as the evaluation of posture in various positions, dyskinesias, muscle tone, range of motion, reflexes, cranial nerve function and sensory function, as well as developmental items, i.e. the items dealing with coordination, fine manipulative abilities and associated movements. The assessment of the developmental

items is not time based, but based on Gestalt evaluation of the quality of performance. The latter is harder than a time-based assessment as it presupposes knowledge on performance that is typical for age.[1] However, it is becoming increasingly clear that the evaluation of the quality of motor behaviour is a powerful and sensitive tool for the evaluation of brain function (Touwen 1978, 1993; Prechtl 1990; Heineman and Hadders-Algra, 2008). Essential to the interpretation of the findings of the neurological assessment are the following notions.

- Single signs have no clinical significance; this holds true even for the isolated presence of a Babinski sign. Neurological signs only have significance when they co-occur with other signs within a functional domain (the 'domain of dysfunction', previously labelled 'cluster of dysfunction'; Hadders-Algra et al, 1988b; Hadders-Algra, 2002).

- Abnormal reflex activity in the absence of other neurological signs has no clinical significance (Nichols and Chen, 1981; Peters et al, 2008).

- The assessment provides information about the neurological profile of the child, thereby providing information about the child's neurological strengths and weaknesses.

- The distinction between the two basic forms of MND: simple MND and complex MND (Hadders-Algra, 2002). This distinction between the two forms is based on age-specific criteria. Until the onset of puberty the distinction is based on the number of domains with a significant dysfunction. In prepubertal children of at least 4 years of age simple MND denotes the presence of one or two domains of dysfunction whereas complex MND denotes the presence of at least three domains of dysfunction. After the onset of puberty the distinction is based on the type of dysfunction present: complex MND denotes the presence of coordination problems or fine manipulative disability; simple MND the presence of other types of dysfunction. The simple form of MND has a high prevalence: it occurs in 15–20% of children. It may be regarded as a form of typical albeit non-optimal brain function (minor neurological *difference*). The complex form of MND occurs in about 5% of children. It is the clinically relevant form of MND as it is clearly linked to prenatal and perinatal adversities and to developmental disorders such as ADHD, autism-spectrum disorders, DCD, dysgraphia, and dyslexia (Hadders-Algra, 2002; Peters et al, 2010; Van Hoorn et al, 2010; De Jong et al, personal communication; Punt et al, 2010). The significance of the neurological profile in terms of MND will be discussed further in Chapter 10.

Intra-observer, inter-observer and test–retest reliability of the assessment of single items is moderate, but good for the various domains of dysfunction and for the classification into simple and complex MND (Peters et al, 2008). As single items have no clinical relevance this means that MND can be assessed reliably.

---

1 Examples of typical performance for the various developmental items are provided on the accompanying DVD.

This technique for the assessment of MND in children and adolescents[2] offers an instrument that enables the examiner to make a refined appraisal of the child's neurological make-up. It is a valuable tool in the work-up of children with learning problems, behavioural disorders, DCD, and speech and language impairment, as detailed knowledge of the child's neurological condition will shed light on the aetiology of the disorder and assist the decision-making necessary to provide therapeutic guidance.

2 The technique may also be used for assessing adults.

Chapter 3

Assessment technique and psychometric properties

Development of the Groningen Assessment

The Groningen Assessment of the child with minor neurological dysfunction (MND) was developed in the 1960s and 1970s (Touwen and Prechtl, 1970; Touwen, 1979). The aim was to develop a comprehensive assessment of neural function. The assessment needs to be reliable in the sense of being replicable by the same and different examiners and it should be based on objective criteria. It should be as complete as possible, but also be applicable in clinical practice. This meant that a compromise was inevitable.

The majority of items included in the assessment deal with motor function, or rather sensorimotor function: posture, muscle tone, reflexes, involuntary movement, coordination, fine manipulative ability, associated movement, and the function of most cranial nerves. A few items address the evaluation of sensory functions: visual acuity, hearing, sense of position, kinaesthesia, and graphaesthesia. Tests that demand a high level of attention from the child, such as the evaluation of light touch, pain, temperature, and two-point discrimination, are not part of the evaluation. However, in individual cases it may be useful to carry out an additional extensive examination of sensory functions.

Over the years some test items have been removed from the examination as they were of little value in determining the presence of domains with significant dysfunction. The following items were removed: following an object with rotation of the trunk while sitting, palmo-mental reflex, Mayer and Léri reflexes, cremasteric reflex, Galant response, examination of the spine while the child is lying, examination of the hip joints, sitting up without the help of hands, fundoscopy, localization of sound (see Touwen, 1979). In addition the item 'pronation and supination with extended arms' is no longer carried out in stance but is included in sitting. When history or examination suggest increased intracranial pressure fundoscopy should be added to the assessment.

Theoretical and technical aspects of the assessment

Developmental approach
The nervous system of a child develops rapidly. Therefore the examiner's approach must be age specific. It is essential for the examiner to be familiar with the developmental processes of motor patterns, sensory mechanisms, cognitive functions, and behavioural expression. The techniques for assessment of MND are adapted to the developing child and his nervous system. This means that this type of examination is based on concepts and techniques fundamentally different from those applied in paediatric neurology which have been extrapolated from adult neurology (Swaiman, 1999; Menkes et al, 2000).

Behavioural state
The behavioural state of the child is an important variable that has a large influence on the results of the examination. The effect of behavioural state on neurological output may be illustrated by the effect of behavioural state on neurological behaviour in young infants. Neurophysiological studies demonstrated that each behavioural state, such as quiet (non-rapid eye movement [REM]) sleep, active (REM) sleep, quiet wakefulness, active wakefulness, and crying, is characterized by a specific neural organization (Prechtl 1972, 1974, 1977; Hadders-Algra et al, 1993). For clinical practice, the notion that the neurophysiological make-up during crying resembles that of mild dysfunction is particularly relevant. Crying is associated with reduced movement variation and less fluent movement (Hadders-Algra et al 1993, Hadders-Algra 2004).

For the assessment of MND this means that an adequate behavioural state is a prerequisite. The child should be assessed while awake and not crying. Moreover, the child should be cooperative, i.e. he should be willing to carry out instructions. Fortunately, children are usually eager to show their abilities so that in general their behavioural state is not a point of concern. However, in the youngest children and in children with behavioural problems it may be more difficult to achieve or maintain an adequate behavioural state and cooperation. In the rare situation that it is totally impossible to achieve an adequate behavioural state the examination should be postponed to another time. Of interest, non-cooperation and refusal during a neurodevelopmental assessment are associated with the presence or emergence of developmental disorders (Langkamp and Brazy, 1999; Wocadlo and Rieger, 2000)

Children with MND frequently are, consciously or unconsciously, aware that they have difficulties with certain tasks. This awareness may induce reluctance to carry out specific tasks. As a result they may openly refuse to perform a task or, more frequently, they may show avoidance behaviour, such as acting like a clown. The recommended strategy is to persist firmly and kindly in asking the child to try the task. Experience allows the examiner to determine whether the child has shown his best performance. It is this best performance which is assessed. It is important that, irrespective of outcome, the attempts of the child to perform the test are rewarded with positive feedback, i.e. with positive comments on effort. Positive feedback is known to be a potent facilitator of a pleasant atmosphere during the examination, in particular in prepubertal children who are more sensitive to positive than to negative feedback (van Duijvenvoorde et al, 2008). However, feedback should be honest. This implies that the examiner should not tell the child that achievements were appropriate if they did not meet age-specific criteria.

The examination has been designed in such a way that it promotes an optimal behavioural state throughout the assessment. For this reason the assessment of cranial nerve function is the last part of the examination. As a good behavioural state is of paramount importance for the interpretation of findings, the presence of a non-optimal behavioural state during certain parts of the examination should be recorded on the assessment form (in the comment boxes of the electronic version of the assessment form on the DVD). Also the presence of other conditions that may affect the findings of the neurological examination, such as fatigue or illness, should be recorded, although undertaking the examination under the latter conditions should be avoided.

Conditions during the assessment
The behavioural state of the child may be affected by environmental conditions and the specifics of the situation. The following points should be taken into account.

DRESSING
In general, children dislike being undressed during an examination. However, the examiner needs an optimal view of the child's motor behaviour, i.e. as little clothing as possible. A good strategy to deal with the conflicting interests of the child and the assessor is to ask the child to bring his gym clothes (without gym shoes). After an introductory conversation with parents and child, the child is asked to put on the gym clothes, for example in the bathroom. This type of clothing allows a proper assessment during most of the examination. The exceptions to this rule are the evaluation of the trunk and the abdominal skin reflex. During these parts of the assessment the child's permission is asked to lift the clothes covering these parts of the body (see Chapter 5, Figure 5.2, p. 54). An optimal view of the child's motor behaviour also requires the absence of socks and shoes, i.e. the child has to be barefoot throughout the assessment.

EXAMINATION ROOM AND EQUIPMENT
Clearly, the room where the examination takes place should be quiet and restful so that the child is not easily distracted and he can feel at ease. Care should be taken to provide a child-friendly atmosphere, which also means that the doctor's paraphernalia, which the child may find frightening, should be removed. In addition, the room and the examiner's hands should be pleasantly warm.

The majority of the assessment is carried out in the sitting and standing position, and during walking. Sitting is evaluated while sitting on a table (Chapters 4 and 8). This implies that sitting is evaluated in a relatively challenging position, as sitting on a table is associated with a lack of support for feet, arms, and back. This challenging position allows for the detection of mild dysfunctions in postural control (Hadders-Algra and Brogren Carlberg, 2008). An examination couch may serve as an alternative for a table as long as it is does not offer support for the feet, arms, and back. A minor part of the assessment is performed in the supine position. This part of the assessment is preferably carried out on a mattress on the floor instead of on an examination couch. Assessing the supine position on the floor has the advantage that it offers a spontaneous situation during which the presence of Gower's sign may be observed (Chapter 7). Assessment of various forms of walking requires some space. When the assessment room is too small for adequate assessment a temporary excursion into the corridor may be the best solution.

To carry out the assessment only a limited amount of equipment is needed for the assessment, i.e. a reflex hammer, a penlight and devices to measure body length, weight, and skull circumference.

PARENTS AND CHILD

The advisability of allowing parents or other familiar adults to be present during the examination has been much disputed. A pragmatic approach is recommended in which the examiner has to keep in mind that the presence of an optimal behavioural state is essential for the assessment of MND. In general, younger children may be more comfortable when a parent is present whereas in older children the presence or absence of a familiar adult matters less.

Usually the assessment is preceded by an interview with both child and parents. This introductory talk gives the child the opportunity to get to know the examiner and get used to the examination room.

It is important that the examination procedure should be playful wherever possible (in the examination of muscle power, for instance) so as to reassure the child. Care should be taken to explain procedures and tests in a clear and standardized way, as children benefit from structure. Therefore it is advisable to count aloud during some tests, such as counting the 20 seconds during which the posture with the arms extended should be kept, counting the number of kicks during kicking, or the number of times the child has placed the tip of the finger on his nose during the finger–nose test. Ideally the relationship between examiner and child resembles that of a dancing couple: the examiner respectfully takes the lead and carefully adapts her movements to those of the child.

Another point that the examiner should consider is that she is likely to tower above the sitting and even the standing child. She should therefore avoid standing over or leaning over the child, but should sit or squat beside, or opposite him.

VIDEO RECORDING

The neurological assessment does not require video recording. Nevertheless, increasingly more people do videotape the assessment. This has the advantage of offering an additional means of documentation. It also allows for supervision and discussion of minor signs with colleagues.

The course of the examination
The examination consists of

(1) an observation of the child's motor behaviour; and
(2) testing of specific nervous functions.

In general, the examiner should keep to the order of the examination as set out in this book. The procedure is divided into several sections. The assessment starts with the child sitting on the table (Chapter 4). This is followed by an examination while the child is standing (Chapter 5). Locomotion (Chapter 6) and a short assessment with the child lying down follows (Chapter 7). The child then returns to the sitting position on the table; in this position sensory functions and the cranial nerves are assessed (Chapter 8). The examination concludes with an assessment of anthropometrics, hand preference, and body schema (Chapter 9). The examiner should allow herself some degree of flexibility within each section and remember that the main aim is to ensure that the child is not disturbed by the examination and remains as happy and responsive as possible. The assessment lasts on average 30 minutes.

The examination's design, aiming at an optimal behavioural state, results in an examination in which the items belonging to a specific domain of dysfunction are scattered throughout the assessment. The neural background of each item is indicated (in the book and on the electronic assessment form on the DVD) by an abbreviation of the domain of dysfunction to which the item belongs (Box 3.1).

Box 3.1 Abbreviations used to indicate specific functional domains

- A, associated movements.
- CN, cranial nerve function.
- Co, coordination and balance.
- F, fine manipulation.
- I, involuntary movements:
  - I-Ath, athetotiform movements
  - I-Ch, choreiform movements
  - I-Tr, tremor.
- PT, posture and muscle tone.
- R, reflexes.
- S, sensory function.

Scoring of items
This method is specifically designed for the detection of MND, and in the discussion of the significance of findings most emphasis is placed on their meaning in the context of MND. However, mention must be made of the significance of findings in relation to more serious conditions, as minor signs may be the first manifestations of a progressive illness. However, as stated earlier, single abnormal signs are rarely of much significance in isolation; signs only have clinical relevance when they co-occur with other signs in the same functional domain.

The majority of items are scored using the trichotomy typical/age-appropriate performance, mildly abnormal, or definitely abnormal. When a child scores mildly or definitely abnormal, it is recommended to record the specifics of the deviant performance on the assessment form (in the comment boxes of the electronic version of the assessment form on the DVD). A definitely abnormal performance is unlikely in children with MND and its presence is an indication for further investigation.

The decision about whether performance is age-appropriate or not is relatively difficult. Criteria for age-specific performance are provided in Chapters 4 to 8. The criteria describe the minimum performance that may be expected at a certain age. In other words, many children perform better than indicated in the criteria used in this book. To facilitate decision-making on the adequacy of performance for age the book includes a DVD with examples of both age-appropriate performance and performance that falls short of this.

At the end of the assessment findings are summarized in the form of dysfunctions per functional domain. Details on the interpretation of findings, including the decision rules for deviant functional domains are discussed in Chapter 10.

Psychometric properties

Reliability
For many years the reliability of the assessment of MND or subtle neurological signs was a matter of concern as most studies concluded that inter-assessor and test–retest agreement was moderate to poor (Werry and Aman, 1976; Shapiro et al, 1978; Holder et al, 1982; Stokman et al, 1986, Vitiello et al, 1989; Kakebeeke et al, 1993). The unsatisfactory reliability, however, can be attributed mainly to the lack of standardized procedures and the lack of criteria for age-specific performance. Therefore, the Groningen Assessment of the child with MND has been updated. It now includes details of standardized procedures and criteria for, and examples of, age-specific performance.

Recently the Groningen Assessment of MND was evaluated in 25 children aged 4–12 years for three types of reliability: intra-assesor, inter-assessor, and test–retest reliability (Peters et al, 2008). The children were assessed by three investigators. Inter- and intra-assessor reliability were based on videotapes of the assessments. To determine test–retest reliability children were reassessed after about 1 month. The study indicated that the three forms of reliability were good for the majority of items and for the trichotomic classification into a normal neurological condition, simple MND, and complex MND ($\kappa = 0.71–0.83$). For most domains of dysfunction reliability was good, but reliability was only moderate for the domains with marked developmental changes, i.e. coordination and fine manipulative ability. The moderate agreement in these two domains emphasizes the need for greater understanding about typical age-specific behaviour. Therefore this book contains information on the criteria for age-specific behaviour and the accompanying DVD contains video examples of performance that is appropriate for age as well as examples of age-inappropriate behaviour.

Validity
Validity is the extent to which an instrument measures what it is intended to measure. The main types of validity are construct validity, concurrent validity, and predictive validity (Tieman et al, 2005).

CONSTRUCT VALIDITY
Construct validity is the extent to which a test reflects the theoretical construct of interest; for the neurological examination the extent to which the neurological condition in terms of MND reflects mild brain dysfunction. The best way to demonstrate construct validity is to study children with and without various forms of MND by means of functional magnetic resonance imaging (MRI) or structural MRI allowing for detailed assessment, such as volumetric MRI or diffusion tensor imaging. But until now such studies have not been performed. One study addressed the relation between the presence of periventricular leukomalacia (PVL) on conventional MRI and a mix of signs of MND and behavioural problems in 8-year-old preterm children, but no relationship between PVL and minor signs could be demonstrated (Olsén et al, 1997). Most information available on construct validity is based on studies of the relationships between MND and the neonatal status of the brain assessed by the newborn's neurological condition or by MRI or ultrasound of the newborn brain. These studies indicated that grade III and IV periventricular haemorrhages and lesions of the white matter and basal ganglia are related to MND at 5 to 6 years, in particular to complex MND (Barnett et al, 2002; Arnaud et al, 2007). The studies of the Groningen Perinatal Project revealed that complex MND is related to the neurological condition of the neonate, whereas simple MND is not (Hadders-Algra et al, 1988b; Soorani-Lunsing, 1993; Hadders-Algra, 2002). Another study indicated that the quality of general movements at 3 months corrected age, which may be regarded as an indicator of the quality of brain function, was related to the presence and severity of MND at 9 to 12 years (Groen et al, 2005). Indirect support for the construct validity of the two basic forms of MND may be derived from studies on relationships between prenatal, perinatal, and neonatal risk factors and the development of MND. These studies indicated that simple MND is associated with preterm birth without serious neonatal complications, severe intrauterine growth retardation without signs of severe fetal compromise, and an Apgar score at 3 minutes below 7 (Ley et al, 1996; Hadders-Algra, 2002; Fallang et al, 2005; Arnaud et al, 2007). It has been hypothesized that these conditions may reflect a situation of stress that may programme the young brain for the development of non-optimal brain function as reflected by the presence of simple MND

(Hadders-Algra, 2003; Schlotz and Phillips, 2009). However, it is important to realize that the large majority of children with simple MND have no history of prenatal, perinatal, or neonatal complications. This makes it likely that the major factor in simple MND may be attributed to genetic information (Hadders-Algra, 2002, 2003). The perinatal developmental studies also revealed a clear relationship between the severity and number of complications in the prenatal, perinatal, and neonatal period and the development of complex MND (Ley et al, 1996; Hadders-Algra, 2002; Fallang et al, 2005; Arnaud et al, 2007). The resemblance of the aetiology of complex MND to that of cerebral palsy, i.e. the association with a chain of pre- and perinatal adversities, gave rise to the suggestion that complex MND, from an aetiological point of view, may be regarded as a borderline form of cerebral palsy (Stanley et al, 2000; Hadders-Algra, 2002, 2003). Interestingly, in about 15% of children with cerebral palsy no abnormalities are found on MRI of the brain (Krägeloh-Mann and Horber, 2007).

CONCURRENT VALIDITY
Concurrent validity is the extent to which scores relate to scores on another measure of the same construct, ideally a criterion standard. If there is no criterion standard available, correlation with other established instruments is assessed. In the domain of MND no criterion standards are available. But the relationships between MND and learning and behavioural disorders could be interpreted as indicators of concurrent (and construct) validity. The studies of the Groningen Perinatal Project (Hadders-Algra et al, 1988a; Soorani-Lunsing et al, 1994; Hadders-Algra 2002; Batstra et al, 2003) demonstrated the following.

- Specific learning disorders, including difficulties in mathematics, reading, and spelling were associated with the presence and severity of MND. Dysfunction in the domains of fine manipulative disability, coordination problems, dysfunctional posture and muscle tone regulation and choreiform dyskinesia in particular play a role in complex MND

- The relationship between behaviour and MND varied with the type of behaviour. Attention problems were strongly related to the presence and severity of MND. The specific domains that played a role were fine manipulative disability, choreiform dyskinesia and – to a lesser extent – coordination problems. Externalizing and internalizing behaviour showed a minor association with neurological make-up. Externalizing behaviour was associated with coordination problems and choreiform dyskinesia, whereas internalizing behaviour was associated with fine manipulative disability.

Other studies indicated that DCD, indicated by poor performance on the Movement ABC or by the presence of dysgraphia, is associated with the presence and severity of MND. Not surprisingly, fine manipulative disability and coordination problems contribute most to the motor problems (Jongmans et al, 1993; Van Hoorn et al, 2010; Peters et al, 2010). A recent study on children with autistism-spectrum disorders (ASD) showed that most children with ASD exhibit complex MND (De Jong et al, personal communication). Studies on the relationship between MND and learning and behavioural problems underscore the notion that 'neurobehavioural relationships' are never one-to-one relationships. Rather the presence and severity of MND should be interpreted as an indicator of the vulnerability of the nervous system to the development of learning and behavioural problems.

PREDICTIVE VALIDITY

Predictive validity is the extent to which scores on the instrument now can predict the outcome in the future on another assessment. The *a priori* expectation in developmental neurology is that perfect correlations between assessments at a young age and those at an older age do not exist, as developmental processes in the brain may be associated with a recovery of dysfunction but also with an emergence of dysfunction (Hadders-Algra, 2004). This is indeed what happens in the development of MND: it may emerge, re-emerge, and disappear. Nevertheless, the data from the Groningen Perinatal Project indicated that children who consistently showed complex MND at an early school age had a considerably higher risk for complex MND in adolescence than children who never or only once showed complex MND (Hadders-Algra, 2002). The significance of the findings from the assessment of MND is considered further in Chapter 10.

Chapter 4

Assessment of the child sitting: part I

Ability to sit

The ability to sit with or without support is recorded. The inability to sit without support indicates the presence of major neurological dysfunction or other serious pathology. The presence of minor neurological dysfunction (MND) does not interfere with the ability to sit without support.

Posture during sitting (PT)[1]

Procedure (Figure 4.1)

The child is asked to sit on a table without the use of arm or elbow support. The child's feet should not touch the floor. The examiner chats with the child so that he is not aware of the fact that the examiner is inspecting the posture of the head, body, and limbs.

Age

Sitting posture can be evaluated from early childhood onwards.

Recording

The posture of head, trunk, arms, and legs is scored separately as follows:

   0 = typical;
   1 = mildly abnormal;
   2 = definitely abnormal.

---

1 See Box 3.1, p. 17 for abbreviations used to indicate specific functional domains.

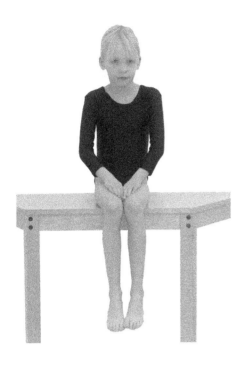

Figure 4.1 The position for the start of the assessment. The child sits on the table; the child's sitting posture is evaluated.

Any persistent deviations from a symmetrical, upright posture are described. Special attention should be paid to the presence of scapulae alatae, a collapsed posture, and asymmetries in the posture of head, trunk, and limbs.

Significance
Children who are slightly hypotonic may sit collapsed and/or on the lower end of the back instead of on the buttocks. This is accentuated when the child is asked to extend his knees and straighten his trunk while supporting himself with his arms. If hypertonia of the hamstring muscles is present, the child adducts his legs during this procedure, which is suggestive of a slight diplegia.

A consistently maintained asymmetrical posture should always arouse a suspicion of pathology, which will be confirmed or dispelled during the rest of the examination.

Deviations as a result of obvious bone or muscle deformities do not need to be mentioned here. A slightly abnormal posture may result from muscular weakness on one or both sides of the body. Lateral incurvations of the trunk may indicate a scoliosis, and this must be checked when the child is standing and lying down.

An asymmetrical posture of the freely hanging legs, often most clearly indicated by the position of the feet, may originate from or be one of the first manifestations of a hemisyndrome. On the other hand, static causes (originating in the hip joint, the ankle, or the foot) must also be borne in mind. Minor asymmetries in the position of the shoulder often occur and have, as a sign on their own, little clinical significance.

Posture with arms extended (PT)

Procedure (Figure 4.2)
The child is asked to stretch out his arms, palms downward, for 20 seconds with eyes closed. The examiner counts the seconds aloud. The test is repeated with the palms turned upward, i.e. with arms outstretched in supination for 20 seconds with eyes closed. During both procedures the hands must be kept apart from each other. Care is taken that the child extends both arms as far as possible. Note that children who have some difficulty with these tasks tend to start with arms in flexion and pronation.

Age
This test is suitable for all children of 4 years and over. Typical performance consists of arm extension without deviation from the starting position.

Recording
(1) Extended arms in pronation is scored as follows:

   0 = typical performance;
   1 = mild unilateral deviation;

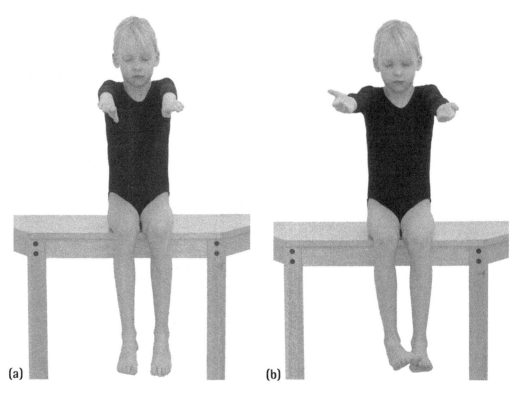

(a)   (b)

Figure 4.2 Posture with arms extended. Typical posture with arms in (a) pronation and (b) supination.

2 = mild bilateral deviation;

3 = marked unilateral deviation;

4 = marked bilateral deviation.

(2) Extended arms in supination is scored as follows:

0 = typical performance;

1 = mild unilateral pronation/flexion/deviation;

2 = mild bilateral pronation/flexion/deviation;

3 = marked unilateral pronation/flexion/deviation;

4 = marked bilateral pronation/flexion/deviation.

During both procedures lateral and vertical deviations from the median line are recorded. During arm extension in supination the degree of pronation and the degree of elbow flexion is also recorded. Asymmetries and the presence of exaggerated effort are noted. The presence of 'spooning', i.e. a relatively high degree of dorsiflexion of the metacarpophalangeal joints, is not taken into account.

Significance
A minor vertical deviation (1–2 cm) is fairly common in children below 6 years of age. The deviation is usually in an upward direction when the arms are pronated and in a downward direction during supination. Children of this age may also show a slight deviation from the median line. However, all such deviations are abnormal in children who are 6 years old and over, and are usually a result of hypotonia where the child may overcorrect the position of the arms, which may cause him to keep the arms below the horizontal (in pronation) or to bring the hands together in the midline (during supination). The deviations are seen in particular during supination. As the eyes are closed during this test, these are purely proprioceptive effects. Mild deviations in muscle tone regulation may be reflected by signs of disproportional effort.

Asymmetries may be the result of a hemisyndrome or some unilateral function disturbance, e.g. sensorimotor innervation disturbance, unilateral coordination difficulties, or local disorders (post-traumatic residual state, muscle, or joint diseases etc.).

Involuntary movements during sitting with and without extended arms (I)

Procedure
Observation of involuntary movements during sitting with and without extended arms.

Age
This test is suitable for all children 4 years old and over. Children below the age of 6 may show athetotiform movements (score 1 or 2). Typical performance in children of at least 6 years is not accompanied by involuntary movements.

Recording
ATHETOTIFORM MOVEMENTS (I-ATH)
These are small slow movements, rather writhing in appearance, which occur quite irregularly and arrhythmically in different muscles. Presumably, they may occur in all muscles of the body, but are seen most easily in the muscles of the fingers and tongue. These are scored as follows:

>   0 = – no athetotiform movements visible, in particular none during arm extension;
>   1 = + 2–5 slow writhing movements during 20-second arm extension;
>   2 = ++ 6–10 writhing movements during 20-second arm extension;
>   3 = +++ continuous writhing movements during 20-second arm extension.

CHOREIFORM MOVEMENTS (I-CH)
These are small, jerky movements that occur irregularly and arrhythmically in different muscles. They may occur in all muscles of the body and can be recorded electromyographically in relaxed muscles when they are not visible on gross inspection. The examiner should look for choreiform movements in fingers, wrist joints (distal choreiform movements) and in the arms and shoulders (proximal choreiform movements; Prechtl and Stemmer, 1962). These are scored as follows:

>   0 = – no choreiform movements visible, in particular none during arm extension;
>   1 = + 2–5 isolated twitches during 20-second arm extension;
>   2 = ++ 6–10 twitches, usually in bursts during 20-second arm extension;
>   3 = +++ continuous twitching during 20-second arm extension.

TREMOR (I-TR)
This consists of involuntary, rhythmical, alternating movements. A clear distinction must be drawn between a resting tremor and tremor that occurs during movements. Here, the resting tremor is recorded. It is worth noting the frequency and regularity of the tremor. These are scored as follows:

>   0 = – no tremor present;
>   1 = + barely discernible tremor;
>   2 = ++ marked tremor of the fingers;
>   3 = ++ marked tremor of the fingers and arms.

Significance
See test of involuntary movements (Chapter 5, p. 56–59).

Mouth-opening and finger-spreading phenomenon (A)

Procedure (Figure 4.3)
The examiner grasps the child's wrists between her thumb and index finger. She extends the child's arms passively and makes sure that the child relaxes wrist and finger joints so that the hands hang down loosely. The examiner then asks the child to open his mouth as wide as he can (phase1), then to close his eyes tightly (phase 2), and finally to stick out his tongue as far as he can (phase 3). Phases 2 and 3 serve to reinforce phase 1.

The test should not be explained in advance to the child, as explanation usually induces confusion and misunderstanding.

Age
This test is suitable for all children of 3 years and over. The degree of associated movement activity during this test shows a large inter-individual variability; the associated activity decreases with increasing age. The following scores (addition of scores from both hands, see below) are considered excessive for age:

- 9 years and over scores >14;
- 11 years and over scores >12; and
- 13 year and over scores >8.

Recording
Spreading and extension of the fingers and thumb may be observed, sometimes accompanied by an extension of the joints of the wrist or of the legs (especially during phases 2 and 3).

Recording is performed in two phases: (1) the actual response, and (2) whether or not the response is appropriate for age.

THE ACTUAL RESPONSE
This is scored as follows:

    0 = no movements of the relaxed finger, wrists, and legs;
    1 = a barely discernible spreading or extension of the fingers;
    2 = a marked spreading and/or extension of the fingers, with some extension of the
         wrists and/or legs;
    3 = maximal spreading and marked extension of the fingers, often accompanied by
         extension of the wrists and/or some extension of the legs.

A score is given for each phase of the test; the final result consists of the sum of the separate scores (a maximum score of 9 for each hand). Each hand is scored separately.

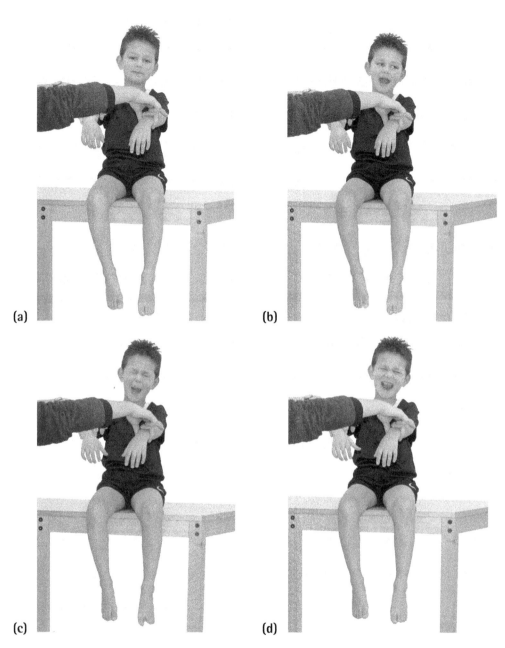

(a)

(b)

(c)

(d)

Figure 4.3 Mouth–opening and finger–spreading phenomenon in a 7–year-old boy.
(a) Starting position: the examiner holds the child's wrists; the child's hands hang down
loosely. (b) Phase 1 of the procedure: opening of the mouth; this child does not show
associated activity in the hands, (c) phase 2: closing of the eyes; this child shows minimal
associated activity in the right hand, reflected by an extension–abduction movement of
the thumb, (d) phase 3: sticking out of the tongue; this child does not show additional
activity in the hands.

FINAL RECORDING
This is scored as follows:

>0 = no associated activity in rest of body;
>
>1 = age-appropriate degree of associated activity;
>
>2 = excessive associated activity.

Significance
The mouth-opening and finger-spreading phenomenon is one of the indicators of the degree of associated movement activity. As an isolated phenomenon test performance has no clinical significance.

Kicking (Co)

Procedure (Figure 4.4)
The examiner holds out her hand on a level midway between the child's knee and ankle at such a distance that the child can easily touch it with his foot. The child is asked to kick the examiner's palm. The test is carried out with the hand in three positions for each foot. First the examiner holds out her hand directly in front of the child's foot then she holds out her hand at a 45° angle to the left and then to the right of the child for three kicks each time.

The examiner takes care that the child does not change sitting position during the sideward kicks. Counting out loud the number of kicks structures the task for the child.

Age
This test is suitable for all children of 4 years and over. Typically developing children are able to hit the examiner's hand three times in each position (nine hits per foot). Children younger than 6 years perform the test considerably more slowly than older children. The youngest children also have a tendency to perseverate.

Recording
This is scored as follows:

>0 = typical performance;
>
>1 = mildly abnormal;
>
>2 = definitely abnormal.

A mild deviancy means that the child occasionally misses the examiner's hand. Performance is scored as definitely abnormal when the child has serious difficulties in hitting the examiner's hand. Asymmetries are recorded.

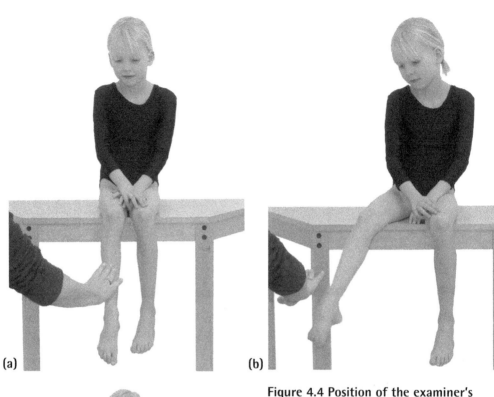

(a)

(b)

Figure 4.4 Position of the examiner's hand during kicking: (a) directly in front of the child's leg, (b) directed outward, at an angle of about 45°, (c) directed inward, at an angle of about 45°.

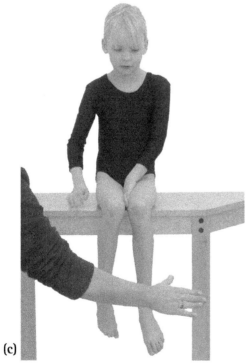

(c)

Significance
Kicking is, like the knee–heel test, a test of the coordination of the legs. Kicking is however considerably easier than the knee–heel test.

Reaction to push against the shoulder while sitting (Co)

Procedure (Figure 4.5)
While the child is sitting upright, with his hand on his knees, and his head centred, the examiner gives a gentle sideward push against the child's shoulder. The upper legs should be in a neutral, i.e. not abducted, position. The ability of the child to remain in a sitting position is recorded. The intensity of the push is graded according to the child's age and body proportions. The examiner should take care to prevent the child from toppling over. To promote the child's feeling of security the examiner holds her arms in a protective way near the child, 'ready to catch' in case the child loses balance.

Age
This test is suitable for all children of 4 years and over, if performed in a playful manner. The child will try to keep balance. In children up to 6 years of age typical performance may include the lifting of the hands from the knees. Older children typically can maintain balance without moving arms and hands.

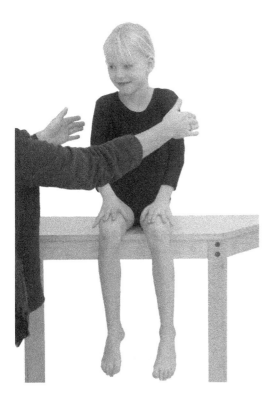

Figure 4.5 Reaction to push against the shoulder while sitting. Note the protective position of the contralateral arm of the examiner.

Recording
The ability to maintain balance and the way the child manages to keep balance are assessed. This is scored as follows:

0 = typical performance;

1 = mildly abnormal;

2 = definitely abnormal.

Mild deviancy means that the child uses more stabilizing arm movements than considered appropriate for age. Performance is scored as definitely abnormal when the child falls sideways and must be caught. Asymmetries are recorded.

Significance
Dysfunctional performance reflects difficulties in trunk coordination and/or balance control.

Assessment of the motor system
The assessment is divided into three parts: active power, resistance against passive movements, and range of movements. Neck, trunk, and hip joints are only assessed in detail when the rest of the assessment has indicated that abnormalities may be present.

Age
The assessment of the motor system is suitable for all children of 4 years and over.

Voluntary relaxation
The child should be relaxed during the assessment of the motor system. Some children find it difficult to relax, which interferes with the assessment. Therefore the degree of voluntary relaxation is recorded as follows:

0 = easy;

1 = difficult;

2 = refuses.

Muscle power

PROCEDURE (FIGURE 4.6)
The child is asked to grasp the examiner's fingers as tightly as possible, using both hands at the same time. The examiner must resist voluntary flexion and extension of the elbow. Abduction and adduction of the arm against resistance provides an estimation of the power of the arm and shoulder muscles. If the examiner suspects the presence of muscle disease pronation and supination should also be tested as, in its early stages, a paresis may manifest itself in the muscles used for these movements (e.g. in muscular dystrophy). The examiner must take hold of the child's hand as if to shake hands and

ask him to pronate and supinate against resistance. Pronation is usually stronger than supination.

If the examiner suspects the presence of muscle disease the strength of the hip and thigh muscles should also be examined at the end of the procedure when the child is lying in supine (for flexion, extension, abduction, and adduction). Flexion and extension of the knee joint and the strength of the ankle and foot movements can be tested while the child is sitting.

The examiner should take care to differentiate between paresis and difficulties in the transformation of a spoken request into a specific movement, i.e. problems in the coordination of motor actions. The two conditions can be distinguished by means of patient and playful repetition of the task: the performance of the child with impaired motor coordination will improve with repetition, that of the child with a paresis will not.

Children in general like to demonstrate muscle power; they put effort into the job; which often is reflected by associated activity in other parts of the body, such as the face.

RECORDING
Muscle power of head, trunk, arms, and legs is scored separately in the following way:

    0 = typical;
    1 = mildly abnormal;
    2 = definitely abnormal.

Asymmetries are recorded.

We believe that the well-known Medical Research Council scale (Medical Research Council, 1978) is not really useful in the case of children with minor dysfunction of the nervous system, since such children are unlikely to exhibit muscular weakness so severe that they are unable to make movements against gravity. Mildly abnormal means that active movements are present, but the child is unable to overcome more than slight resistance (MRC partially 3 and 4); definitely abnormal means that no active movements can be performed (MRC 0, 1, 2, and partially 3).

SIGNIFICANCE
Decreased active power may result from neuromuscular disease, paresis, or general weakness or it could be a symptom of an infectious disease, a metabolic disturbance, or malnutrition. Box 4.1 provides a review of the main causes of neuromuscular weakness in childhood. A detailed discussion is beyond the scope of this book. A slight decrease in muscle strength may be the first manifestation of a progressive disorder, and cases of unilateral decrease should be noted with particular care. The examiner must try to discover whether the muscle weakness had a central or peripheral origin. It should be remembered that a central paresis in young children need not be accompanied by an

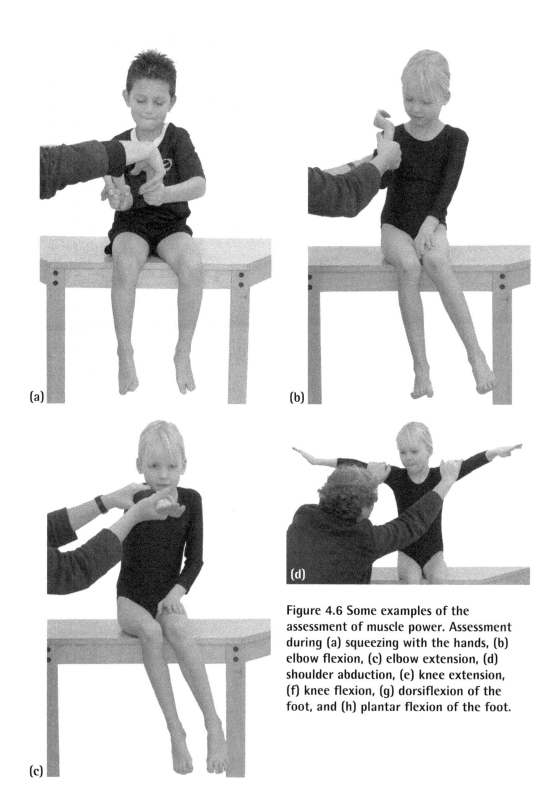

(a)

(b)

(c)

(d)

Figure 4.6 Some examples of the assessment of muscle power. Assessment during (a) squeezing with the hands, (b) elbow flexion, (c) elbow extension, (d) shoulder abduction, (e) knee extension, (f) knee flexion, (g) dorsiflexion of the foot, and (h) plantar flexion of the foot.

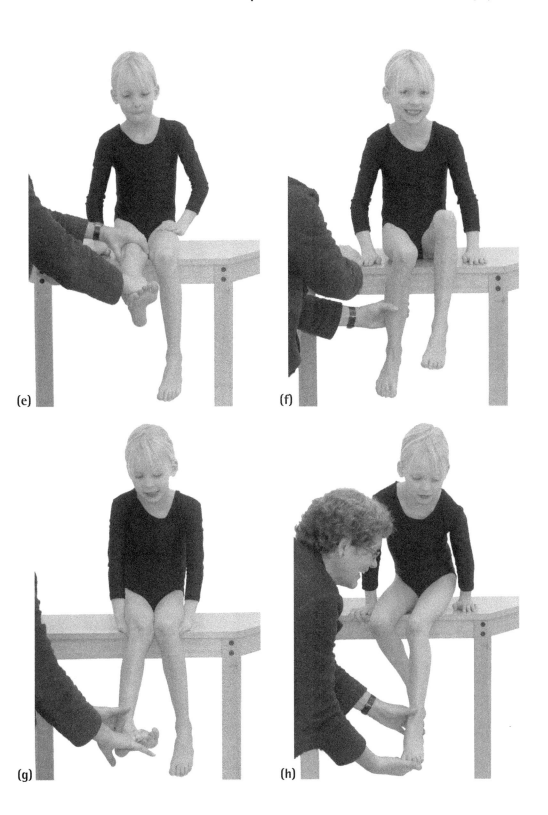

(e)

(f)

(g)

(h)

increased resistance to passive movements. Usually, the results of the assessment of the tendon reflexes and to exteroceptive responses (e.g. plantar response) will help to differentiate between central, peripheral, and myogenic weakness.

Box 4.1 Common causes of non–acute neuromuscular weakness in childhood (based on Malik and Painter, 2004)

- Disorders of the central nervous system e.g.
  - cerebral palsy;
  - metabolic disorders, such as leukodystrophies or mucopolysaccharidosis;
  - chromosomal abnormalities, such as Down syndrome.
- Metabolic, nutritional, endocrine e.g.
  - organic acidaemias;
  - hypercalcaemia;
  - hypothyroidism.
- Spinal cord disorders.
- Juvenile spinal muscular atrophies.
- Neuropathies.
- Myasthenic syndromes.
- Myopathies.
- Connective tissue disorders.

Resistance against passive movements (PT)

PROCEDURE (FIGURE 4.7)
The child is asked to relax as much as possible, and resistance is tested and assessed by passively moving the various joints. The shoulder joint is tested by holding the shoulder girdle firm with one hand and moving the child's upper arm through the range of movements of the shoulder joint with the other hand. To test the elbow, the upper arm is held firm while the lower arm is flexed and extended; to test the wrist joint, the lower arm is held firm in a semi-flexed position (to avoid pronation and supination that is tested separately) and the hand is moved.

While the child is sitting, the position of the hip joint can be standardized by holding the upper leg firm, so that resistance of the knee can be tested. To test the ankle joint, the lower leg is held firm with the knee is a semi-flexed position.

The passive movements must be carried out slowly and carefully, and should be repeated several times.

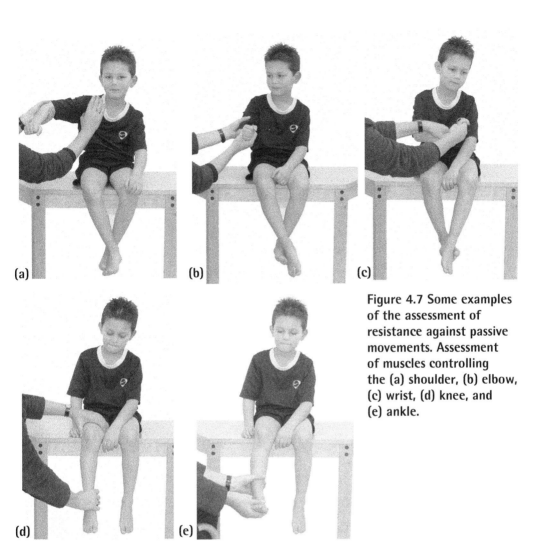

(a)

(b)

(c)

Figure 4.7 Some examples of the assessment of resistance against passive movements. Assessment of muscles controlling the (a) shoulder, (b) elbow, (c) wrist, (d) knee, and (e) ankle.

(d)

(e)

RECORDING

Resistance against passive movements of head, trunk, arms, and legs is recorded separately as follows:

0 = typical;

1 = mildly abnormal:

somewhat weak resistance, mild hypotonia (↓)

somewhat strong resistance, mild hypertonia (↑)

resistance irregularly varying between somewhat weak and somewhat

strong, mildly varying muscle tone; (↕)

2 = definitely abnormal:

weak resistance, marked hypotonia (↓↓)

strong resistance, marked hypertonia (↑↑)

resistance irregularly varying between weak and strong, marked varying muscle tone.(↕↕).

SIGNIFICANCE

Generally speaking, a child's resistance to passive movements depends to a certain degree on his soma type and muscle bulk. Girls often show a level of resistance to passive movements which, while typical for them, would be considered low in boys.

A thorough discussion of the cause of increased and decreased resistance against passive movements is beyond the scope of this book, which is principally concerned with minor, often inconspicuous, deviations from optimal functioning. Nevertheless, the examiner must bear in mind that in extreme cases, a slight variation in resistance to passive movements may be one of the first signs of a progressive disorder of the neuromuscular system (e.g. leukodystrophies, cerebroretinal degenerations, dyskinesias such as Huntington chorea, cerebral neoplasms, or toxic degenerations such as lead poisoning).

It should be noted that disturbances of the afferent input to the spinal cord (afferent nerves, spinal ganglion, dorsal roots, or dorsal columns) may result in a decreased resistance to passive movements before other signs are present. In cases of hypotonia, not all muscles are necessarily involved at the same time. One may be impaired whereas others function normally, e.g. the peroneal muscle of the lower leg (see test for walking on heels, Chapter 6, p. 86).

A decreased resistance against passive movements is often found in children with learning disability. In children with MND mild hypotonia and mildly varying muscle tone are more often found than mild hypertonia. In case of mild hypertonia specific attention should be paid to the presence of more focal neurological signs; which are more compatible with a specific neurological diagnosis, such as a mild unilateral spastic cerebral palsy.

Mildly variable muscle tone regulation, i.e. a condition in which muscle tone irregularly changes from mild hypotonia to mild hypertonia, is seen particularly in children born preterm. The pathophysiological background of this phenomenon is unknown. It is conceivable that it is the more 'mature' form of the MND that during infancy is expressed as 'transient dystonia'. (Drillien, 1972; Sommerfelt et al, 1998; De Vries and De Groot, 2002).

It is also beyond the scope of this book to discuss the differentiation between spasticity, 'lead-pipe' rigidity, and 'cog-wheel' rigidity, since these phenomena evidently surpass the bounds of MND. An increased resistance to passive movements, if not of central nervous system origin, may be the result of myogenic (scleroderma, acute myositis) or articular (acute or chronic rheumatoid arthritis) disorders. Conclusions about the origin and diagnosis in an individual patient can only be made when the examination has been completed.

Range of passive movements

PROCEDURE
In testing resistance in passive movements, the joints are moved through their full range, and hyperextensibility or limitation of movements is recorded. The range of movements shows wide individual variation. However, the average range of movements for the various joints are given below (Wu et al, 2002, 2005).

Head
- Anteflexion: the chin can touch the chest.
- Retroflexion: an imaginary plane from mentum to occiput approaches the horizontal.
- Rotation: 70°, each side.

Shoulder
- Abduction: to ±110° with shoulder girdle held firm.
- Anteflexion: to ±100° with shoulder girdle held firm.
- Retroflexion: to ±60° with shoulder girdle held firm.
- Other movements are not considered.

Elbow
- Extension/flexion: 0°–0°–±150°, depending on the thickness of the arm.

Wrist
- Extension/flexion: 70°–0°–90°.

Knee
- Extension/flexion: 15°–0°–130°, depending on the bulk of the leg.

Ankle
- Plantar flexion/dorsal flexion: 45°–0°–20°.

RECORDING
Only the degree of deviation from the average range of movements described above is recorded, and this is quantified as far as is possible by using, for example a goniometer. Asymmetries are noted.

The range of passive movements of head, trunk, arms, and legs is recorded separately as follows:

0 = typical;

1 = mildly abnormal:

mild limitation ($\downarrow$)

mild hyperextensibility ($\uparrow$);

2 = definitely abnormal:

marked limitation ($\downarrow\downarrow$)

marked hyperextensibility ($\uparrow\uparrow$).

SIGNIFICANCE

The range of movements of the joints may vary considerably from child to child, especially with regard to the degree of extension. Slender girls have wider ranges of movements than more heavily built boys of the same age. The ethnic background should also be noted, as for example children of Asian or Eurasian parents often show a greater range of movements than white children of the same age.

An abnormal increase in the range of movements is generally related to a low resistance against passive movements. Limitation of movements may originate in the ligaments of the joints, the muscles, or the motor neurons. Complaints of pain during the examination should be very carefully investigated. Testing the range of movements may be painful, particularly where there are articular or myogenic limitations of movement, and this pain may in turn cause further limitation of movements during the examination. Spontaneous pain caused by acute arthritis or dermomyositis, for example, or even from any other origin, may decrease the range of movements by causing an inability to relax the musculature, thus interfering with the optimal range of movements present. Persistent asymmetries should always be carefully considered, since they may be part of a hemisyndrome. This conclusion can only be made on completion of the entire examination, when other causes (e.g. local or peripheral) can be excluded.

Examination of reflexes

General remarks

During the elicitation of reflexes, the posture of the arms and legs should be symmetrical and the child's head should be centred in the midline, in order to avoid the differential influences of asymmetric postures (especially of the head and trunk) on the test results.

Typically, reflex activity is variable (Stam and Van Crevel, 1989). This means that at least five reflex taps are required to determine the average intensity and threshold of a reflex. Abnormal responses are characterized by a stereotyped low or high intensity and/or a stereotyped low or high threshold.

Age
Reflex activity can be assessed at any age. Children of 4 years and over typically do not exhibit a dorsiflexion of the big toe during the footsole reaction and do not show a plantar grasp reaction.

Biceps reflex (R)

PROCEDURE (FIGURE 4.8)
The child is asked to put his flexed arms on his lap so that the elbows are in a neutral position. The examiner ascertains for herself that the elbow joints are relaxed by gently moving the child's forearms. She places a finger on the tendon of the child's biceps muscle, and gives a short tap on this finger with the reflex hammer. If no response is obtained, the degree of flexion of the elbow must be varied until the position that gives the best response is achieved. The test should be repeated with taps of varying intensity in order to evaluate the reflex threshold. By keeping the position of the arms symmetrical during the elicitation of the reflex the results on both sides can be compared directly.

RESPONSE
A quick flexion of the elbow, caused by the contraction of the biceps muscle, may be seen and/or felt. Often the brachialis muscle also contracts and the response (flexion of the forearm) is more evident. If the brachialis radialis muscle (situated at the radial site of the forearm and the biceps tendon) is stimulated, a slight pronation of the forearm may occur. Many children show a gentle flexion of the fingers, especially if the forearm is kept supinated; however, this response, which means a spreading of the stimulus to other muscles, is not necessarily present. Sometimes, however, a slight flexion of the fingers is the only response to be observed, especially in children with biceps reflexes of low intensity. In this case we interpret the flexion of the fingers as a positive response of low intensity of the biceps reflex, but only if the position of the elbow joint is sufficiently varied to guarantee that no better response can be obtained.

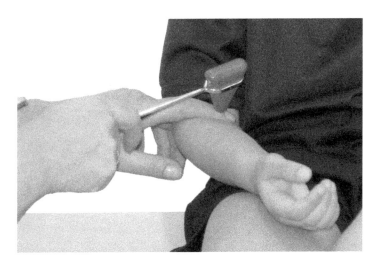

Figure 4.8 Technique for the biceps reflex: the arm of the child rests in relaxed semi-flexion of the elbow: the examiner puts an index finger on the child's biceps tendon and taps with the reflex hammer on her own finger.

41

RECORDING
Performance is scored as follows:

> 0 = typical response
> 1 = abnormal:
>> absent response (noted in comment box)
>> weak response, the response is felt but not seen (↓)
>> exaggerated response: sometimes a few clonic beats; generally a marked flexion of the fingers whether the forearm is kept supinated or not (↑).

Asymmetries are noted.

Triceps reflex (R)

PROCEDURE (FIGURE 4.9)
The examiner takes the child's wrist in one hand so that the elbow is semi-flexed, and confirms that the elbow and shoulder muscles are relaxed by gently moving these joints. She taps with the reflex hammer on the tendon of the triceps muscle about 1 to 2 cm above the olecranon. The test should be repeated with taps of varying intensity on the tendon and muscle at a greater distance from the olecranon, in order to evaluate the reflex threshold.

RESPONSE
A quick, slight extension of the elbow caused by contraction of the triceps muscle may be observed.

Figure 4.9 Technique for the triceps reflex: the examiner gently holds the child's arm in semi-flexion; when she senses that the arm is relaxed, the triceps tendon is tapped.

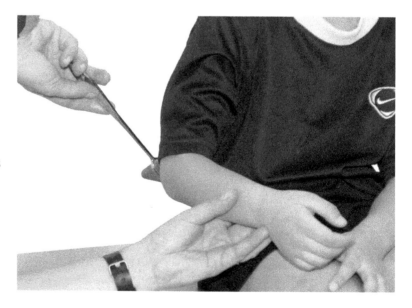

RECORDING
Performance is scored as follows:

> 0 = typical response;
> 1 = abnormal:
>> absent response (noted in comment box)
>> weak response, the response is felt but not seen (↓)
>> exaggerated response: clonic beats are only very rarely found; sometimes a slight extension of the fingers (↑).

Asymmetries are noted.

Knee jerk (R)

PROCEDURE (FIGURE 4.10)
The examiner positions herself low down in front of the child, and takes the child's leg in one hand, making sure that the knee joint is relaxed by gentle moving the leg. She keeps the knee in a semi-flexed position, and gives a short tap with the reflex hammer on the patellar tendon ±1 cm below the patella. It is important to check the spot, as a tap slightly to the side of the tendon will often result in a poor response. If no response is obtained, the examiner changes the degree of flexion of the knee joint until she finds the position that gives the best result. If a positive response is obtained, the examiner varies the intensity of the tap and the distance from the patella (on or below the

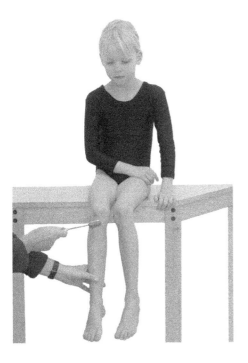

Figure 4.10 Technique for the knee jerk: the examiner gently holds the lower leg of the child; when she senses that the leg is relaxed, the patellar tendon is tapped.

insertion of the quadriceps tendon at the tibia) and above the patella on the muscle itself, in order to evaluate the reflex threshold.

RESPONSE
A quick extension of the knee, caused by contraction of the quadriceps muscle, may be observed. Younger children may also show a slight adductor contraction, generally in the opposite leg, but occasionally in both legs. The presence of any adductor contraction should be recorded separately for each side.

RECORDING
Performance is scored as follows:

> 0 = typical response;
> 1 = abnormal:
>> absent response (noted in comment box)
>> weak response, the response is felt but not seen ($\downarrow$)
>> exaggerated response, sometimes followed by a few clonic beats and/or adduction of the opposite and/or stimulated leg ($\uparrow$).

Asymmetries are noted.

Ankle jerk (R)

PROCEDURE (FIGURE 4.11)
The examiner holds the child's foot and keeps it in a neutral position in relation to the child's leg so that she can control the degree of relaxation by slightly moving the foot and leg. Using a reflex hammer, the examiner taps on the Achilles tendon about 2–3 cm above the insertion at the calcaneus (Figure 4.11a). If there is no response, she should vary the relative positions of the ankle joint. If a positive response is obtained, the examiner repeats the tap a number of times, varying the intensity of the tap and varying the distance from the insertion of the tendon. In this way she can evaluate the reflex threshold.

In case a tap readily elicits a response the presence of ankle clonus is assessed. The examiner grasps the child's forefoot (palm at the plantar side, thumb on the dorsum of the foot) and produces a brisk and sudden dorsiflexion of the foot (Figure 4.11b). As a result clonic beats may follow.

The common technique for the elicitation of the ankle jerk in adults, which consists of asking the patient to kneel on a chair or table with the feet dangling, is usually of no use with children, as they do not relax easily in that position.

RESPONSE
A brief plantar flexion of the foot at the ankle may be observed. In nervous children it is sometimes accompanied by a slight flexion of the knees and/or toes.

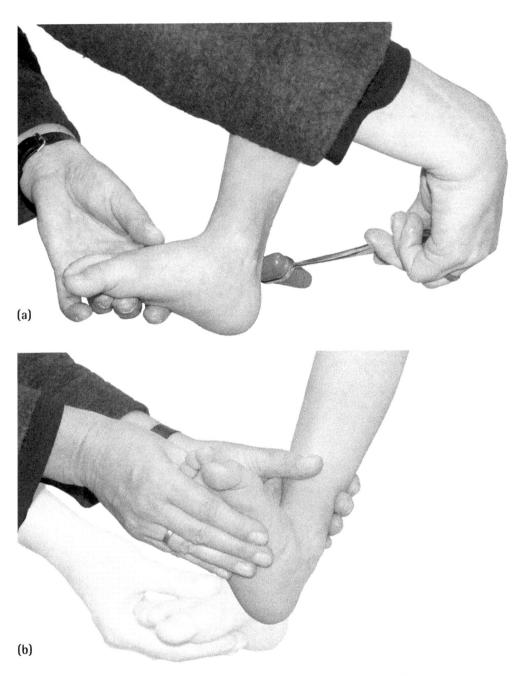

(a)

(b)

Figure 4.11 Technique for the ankle jerk and ankle clonus. (a) Ankle jerk: the examiner gently holds the child's foot with the ankle in a neutral position; when she senses that the ankle and foot are relaxed the Achilles tendon is tapped. (b) Ankle clonus: the examiner holds the child's foot in her hand and produces a brisk and sudden dorsiflexion of the foot.

RECORDING
Performance is scored as follows:

> 0 = typical response;
> 1 = abnormal:
>> absent response (noted in comment box)
>> weak response, the response is felt but not seen (↓)
>> exaggerated response, sometimes followed by a few clonic beats or sustained clonus (↑).

Asymmetries are noted.

Threshold of tendon reflexes

As each reflex is tested, the intensity of the stimulus in the individually standardized position is varied. If the reflex response is found to be of high intensity or if a weak stimulus is sufficient to elicit a response, the extent of the area from which the reflex is elicitable is explored further. Although there is a difference between a low threshold (evaluated by taps of varying intensity) and the extension of the reflexogenic area (evaluated by tapping at varying distances from the original spot), these two are so closely correlated that for practical purposes they are considered comparable.

The examiner sometimes faces the problem of deciding how many trials should be made before the reflex can be considered absent. If no reflex response has been elicited after about 10 trials in a good standardized neutral position with stimuli of varying intensity, and the child's muscles are quite relaxed, then an 'absent response' can be recorded.

RECORDING
Performance is scored as follows:

> 0 = typical threshold;
> 1 = abnormal:
>> no reflex elicitable (noted in comment box)
>> high threshold, high intensity of stimulus necessary (↑)
>> low threshold, very low intensity of stimulus necessary; extension of area from which reflex is elicitable (↓).

Asymmetries are noted.

SIGNIFICANCE
Absence of reflexes or low-intensity reflexes with a high threshold may be a sign of a muscle disease, a peripheral nervous disorder, or a lower or upper motor neuron disease. An exaggerated response may be because of a lesion or dysfunction of upper motor neurons. A high-intensity reflex is quite often correlated with a low threshold, although this is not inevitable. Children with MND may have a low threshold for a reflex of normal intensity. The reverse may also be found.

Asymmetries require further investigation, as in combination with other signs they may originate from a hemisyndrome. Obvious asymmetries of tendon reflex responses may sometimes be present as an isolated finding, and they may or may not be of clinical significance. It is possible that one asymmetrical reflex may be the first, or even the only, manifestation of a peripheral nervous disorder or a local muscle disease. It may also be the residual effect of a past disorder (traumata, infectious diseases with high fever, disorders of endocrine gland function). Consistent asymmetries in thresholds only and asymmetries without an obvious lateralized pattern may be signs of MND. Where laterality is well established (especially in 5- to 7-year-old children), a slight asymmetry of the threshold for tendon reflexes may be found but need not be clinically significant. The low threshold most often occurs on the side of the arm or leg of preference.

Plantar response or footsole response (R)

PROCEDURE (FIGURE 4.12)
The examiner holds the child's foot steady in a neutral position and scratches along the lateral side of the sole from the toes towards the heel with the point of a sharp object or her thumbnail. The stimulus should be a relatively slow, firm scratch, but not strong enough to elicit a withdrawal of the leg. This technique is rather different from the classical test of the plantar response, whereby the examiner scratches along the lateral side of the sole towards the toes. That method has the drawback of terminating with the specific stimulus for the plantar grasp reaction: thus, a plantar flexion of the toes in this instance may indicate either a positive grasp reaction or a plantar response. Clearly, it is

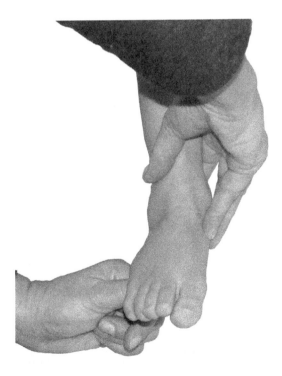

Figure 4.12 Technique for the footsole reaction: the examiner holds the child's ankle and scratches along the lateral side of the sole from the toes towards the heel with the point of a sharp object or the nail of the thumb. Here a typical response is observed: a slight plantar flexion of the big toe.

important to differentiate between the two, especially as a positive grasp reaction in a 4-year-old may be a manifestation of a delay in maturation of the central nervous system.

RESPONSE
Four different qualities of response in the big toe may be observed.

(1) A negative response; no movement of the toe as a result of the stimulus.
(2) A tonic plantar flexion of the big toe.
(3) A jerky and variable dorsi- or plantar flexion of the big toe.
(4) A tonic, stereotyped dorsiflexion of the big toe.

In the other toes spreading or fanning may be present.

RECORDING
Performance is scored as follows:

> 0 = typical: responses: 1 to 3 above;
>
> 1 = abnormal: presence of a tonic, stereotyped dorsiflexion of the big toe, i.e. Babinski sign (response 4 above; ↑).

Asymmetries are recorded.

SIGNIFICANCE
Although the optimal response is plantar flexion, in clinical practice a 'no reaction' score may also be considered as falling within the optimal range. Inconsistent dorsiflexion is frequently seen in children, especially in the younger age range. The response usually has a jerky quality. However, if this jerky dorsiflexion is clearly stereotyped it should be considered abnormal. Variable jerky dorsiflexion may be caused by the child's ticklishness (perhaps a result of tension and nervousness) and is usually of no clinical significance. Sustained, stereotyped dorsiflexion, which does not originate from a foot deformity (pes cavus), reflects a neurological dysfunction, especially if other signs of neurological dysfunction are also present. In the case of pes cavus, the misleading dorsiflexion of the big toe can often be overcome by pushing up the head of the first metatarsal bone. The movement of the big toe (and of the other toes) in the plantar response results from the interplay between foot extensors and flexors. In infants and young toddlers there is a shift of balance between flexors and extensors that favours dorsiflexion and spreading of the toes, whereas in children of 3 years and over the cooperation between extensors and flexors usually leads to plantar flexion of the toes or and an 'indifferent' response (no movements or change of posture whatsoever). When there are foot deformities, the equilibrium between extensors and flexors may again be shifted (for example, towards the dorsiflexed side in pes cavus). Although the disturbance of equilibrium may be overcome by correcting the posture of the foot, the correcting manoeuvre may elicit a grasp response, particularly in toddlers, in which case a clear differentiation of the ultimate movement of the big toe remains problematic (e.g. Friedrichs or Marie-Hoffmans disease).

Fanning or spreading of the toes is often present in children aged 5 years or less, but in older children it can be a sign of neurological dysfunction, i.e. when it is not part of a general withdrawal movement of the leg.

Asymmetries may be of great significance and require further investigation. Slight differences between the responses of the left and right foot, such as plantar flexion on one side and a negative response on the other, may be regarded as meaningful asymmetries if other slight signs of lateralization are also present. An isolated asymmetry, i.e. an asymmetry of the plantar responses without other signs of minor dysfunction, is usually of no clinical significance.

Plantar grasp reaction (R)

PROCEDURE (FIGURE 4.13)
The examiner places her index finger against the heads of the metatarsal bones, approaching them from the lateral side of the foot, and presses firmly.

RESPONSE
Plantar flexion of all toes may be observed.

RECORDING
Performance is scored as follows:

    0 = absent, or minimal, inconsistent response;
    1 = present, i.e. sustained response for approximately 10 seconds.

Asymmetries are recorded.

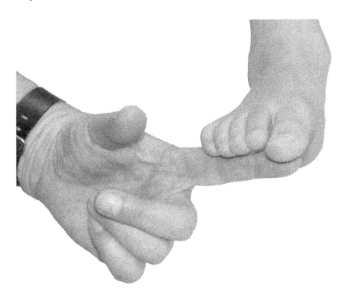

Figure 4.13 Plantar grasp reaction: the examiner's finger is pressed against the heads of the metatarsal bones, approaching them from the lateral side of the foot. Here: no response.

SIGNIFICANCE

A sustained response is always abnormal. It may merely be a sign of developmental delay or it may be a manifestation of central nervous system damage. When there is severe deterioration in the functioning of the central nervous system the grasp reflex may reappear; however, this eventuality surpasses the bounds of MND.

Chapter 5
Assessment of the child standing

Ability to stand

The ability to stand with or without help is recorded. The inability to stand without support indicates the presence of major neurological dysfunction or other serious pathology. The presence of minor neurological dysfunction (MND) does not interfere with the ability to stand without support.

Posture during standing, including inspection of the trunk (PT)

Procedure (Figure 5.1)

The child stands relaxed with arms hanging loosely by his side. The examiner inspects the posture of the head, trunk, and limbs. The examiner should also carefully inspect the spine and the skin of the trunk.

Special attention should be paid to possible lateral incurvation of the spine (i.e. scoliosis). When scoliosis is suspected, the forward-bending test may be applied, even though it should be recognized that a negative test does not preclude the presence of scoliosis (Karachalios et al, 1999).

Age

Standing posture can be evaluated from early childhood onwards.

Recording

The posture of head, trunk, arms and legs is scored separately as follows:

> 0 = typical;
>
> 1 = mildly abnormal;
>
> 2 = definitely abnormal.

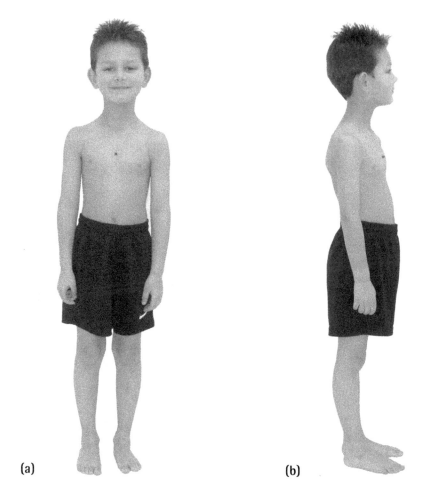

(a) (b)

Figure 5.1 Assessment of posture in stance: (a) frontal and (b) lateral view. Typical posture of a 7-year-old boy.

Any persistent deviations from a symmetrical, upright posture are described. Special attention should be paid to the presence of scapulae alatae, kyphosis, exaggerated lumbar lordosis, scoliosis, and persistent asymmetries in limb posture.

Significance
There is marked variation in body posture. Round shoulders are often of no neurological significance. A kyphosis and exaggerated lumbar lordosis can result from static defects or from a generalized muscular hypotonia (except in the case of slender young girls, who often show exaggerated lumbar lordosis without any neurological defect).

Asymmetry may be part of a hemisyndrome involving the trunk and/or extremities. In the case of scoliosis, a skeletal anomaly should be suspected, although it may originate from a unilateral muscular weakness (poliomyelitis) or from hypertonia (irritative processes, myositis, intercostal neuritis, renal neoplasm). A paediatric examination is often necessary to exclude the possibility of internal diseases. There is a possibility that, in very rare cases, scoliosis may be one of the first manifest signs of Friedrichs ataxia.

Some degree of genu valgum and pes valgus under 6 years of age is usual, and is accompanied by walking and standing on the instep of the foot. The child may thus give the impression of being flat footed, but if the ankle joint is corrected or the child is asked to stand on tiptoes, the arch often turns out to be sufficient (presence of 'flexible flat foot'). The posture of the feet varies widely among typically developing children, one reason being because of variation in the laxity of the ligaments of the joints. Extreme genu valgum and/or pes valgus may sometimes have a neurological cause (hypotonia), especially in children older than about 6 years. It is essential to differentiate between flat feet (pes planus) and standing on the instep (associated with broad forefeet). The latter is often a sign of hypotonia, whereas flat feet are usually of no neurological significance. An extensive discussion about pes cavus and other foot deformities, which accompany severe neurological diseases, falls outside the scope of this book. It is well known that pes cavus may be one (or even the only) manifestation of a spinal dysraphism, and on rare occasions it may be the first sign of Friedrichs ataxia or an inherited motor and sensory neuropathy.

The skin along the midline of the back is worth particularly careful inspection. A naevus, dimple, hairy patch or small lipoma may be the only external signs of an underlying spina bifida occulta. Naevi found laterally from the midline and often in a dermatomic area of the skin (café-au-lait spots) or small fibromas, etc. may arouse the suspicion of Recklinghausen disease before the appearance of other symptoms. The naevi vasculosi, which accompany Sturge-Weber disease, may be present on the skin of the back when they are not very conspicuous in the trigeminal area of the face; more often, they are not confined just to the skin of the back. Café-au-lait spots, combined with white (vitiligo) spots and sebaceous adenomas (often only pinpoint size), may be a sign of tuberous sclerosis before the disease is clinically evident. Sometimes a sebaceous adenoma is the only sign of disease, and it may be present for many years without other symptomatology.

Abdominal skin reflex (R)

Procedure (Figure 5.2)
The examiner scratches with a pin or a fingernail (e.g. nail of the little finger) from the side of the abdominal wall towards the centre, above and below the navel. We prefer a standing position, as experience has shown that a lying child tends to contract his abdominal muscles. Sometimes it is worthwhile to distract the child by talking to him or drawing his attention to some surrounding object in order to obtain full relaxation of his abdominal muscles.

Figure 5.2 Abdominal skin reflex: the examiner scratches with a pin or a fingernail (e.g. nail of the little finger) from the side of the abdominal wall towards the centre, above (as shown in the figure) and below the navel.

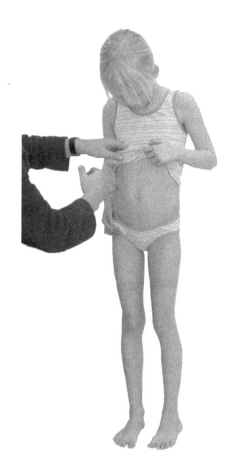

The response to this exteroceptive reflex may diminish after two or more trials. If several trials are needed to determine the nature, in particular the symmetry, of the response, there should be an interval (sometimes lasting a few minutes) between each trial.

Age
The abdominal skin reflex can be assessed at any age.

Response
There should be a contraction of the abdominal muscles in the stimulated area. In children who are obese the contraction may be hardly visible.

Recording
This is scored as follows:

> 0 = symmetrically present;
> 1 = unilaterally absent;
> 2 = bilaterally absent.

Significance
Absence of the abdominal skin reflex may be because of spinal dysfunction at the segmental levels of the reflex (T7–L1); a supraspinal lesion may modify the excitability of the spinal centre of the reflex. However, depression or absence may well be as a result of non-neurological causes (e.g. acute surgical problems, distended bladder, surgical scarring of the skin, strong distension of the abdominal muscles caused by ascites).

The abdominal skin reflex should be symmetrical; asymmetries may be of significance if other lateralized signs in the same left/right pattern occur.

Romberg test (Co)

Procedure (Figure 5.3)
The child is asked to keep his eyes closed for 10 to 15 seconds. With very young children it may be necessary to invent a game, e.g. 'Let's see how long you can stand still with your eyes closed. Close your eyes and I shall count how long you can do it for.' To promote the child's feeling of security the examiner holds her arms in a protective way near the child, 'ready to catch' in case the child loses balance.

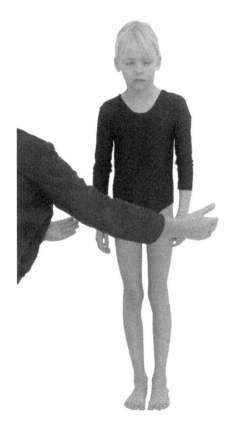

Figure 5.3 Posture during Romberg test, i.e. standing with eyes closed. Note the protective posture of the examiner's arms.

Age
This test is suitable for all children of 4 years and over. Children aged less than 6 often need a few movements of ankles and toes to maintain balance without any actual displacement of the feet.

Recording
As this is a test of balance, i.e. the ability to maintain equilibrium without visual control, the amount of movement of the trunk, arms, legs, and feet needed for this purpose is recorded as follows:

> 0 = typical, stands still/only moves ankles or toes;
> 1 = mildly abnormal, shows trunk and arm movements;
> 2 = definitely abnormal, loses balance.

A consistent tendency to fall to one side should be recorded.

Significance
Slight swaying movements of the body unaccompanied by isolated arm or leg movements are often seen – these movements are inherent to proper postural control (Latash and Hadders-Algra, 2008).

Involuntary movements may interfere with optimal performance and this should be taken into account in the final interpretation of the findings.

A tendency to fall to one side may be a sign of unilateral vestibular or cerebellar dysfunction. A lack of balance without consistent laterality often reflects delayed or dysfunctional postural control. It may also be caused by muscular weakness or intensive dyskinesia.

Test for involuntary movements (I)

General remarks
The words athetoid and athetotic are extremely misleading; sometimes they are used synonymously and sometimes they are given distinct meanings. The Groningen 'school' has attempted here to give a precise operational definition of what is understood by certain terms in each instance. When more than one term is used synonymously in the literature alternatives are listed with the notion that many authors have been imprecise in their use of such terms. The fact that one type of movement shows some resemblance to another type of movement does not mean that both types of movement are aetiologically or pathogenetically identical e.g. choreatic and choreiform movements.

Procedure (Figure 5.4)
The child is asked to stand with the feet placed less than 2 cm apart and the head centred, and then to stretch out both arms with the fingers spread as wide apart as

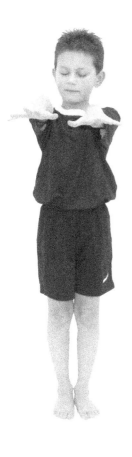

Figure 5.4 Posture during test for involuntary movements. The child stands for 20 seconds with extended arms in pronation, the fingers spread as wide apart as possible and eyes closed.

possible, and to close his eyes. The child is requested to keep the arms still in space for 20 seconds. The hands must be kept apart from each other during the entire test. The examiner counts the seconds out loud.

Age
The test is difficult to carry out with children less than 4 years old. From 4 years onwards children can comply with the test however, those below the age of 6 may show athetotiform movements (score 1 or 2). Typical performance in children of at least 6 years is not accompanied by involuntary movements.

Recording

CHOREIFORM MOVEMENTS (CHOREATIC MOVEMENTS; I-CH)
These are small, jerky movements, which occur irregularly, and arrhythmically in different muscles. They may occur in all muscles of the body and can be recorded electromyographically in relaxed muscles when they are not visible on gross inspection. The examiner should look for choreiform movements in fingers, wrist joints (distal choreiform movements), and in the arms and shoulders (proximal choreiform movements) (Prechtl and Stemmer, 1962). These are scored as follows:

> 0 = – no choreiform movements visible, in particular none during arm extension;
> 1 = + 2–5 isolated twitches during 20-second arm extension;
> 2 = ++ 6–10 twitches, usually in bursts during 20-second arm extension;
> 3 = +++ continuous twitching during 20-second arm extension.

Distal and proximal choreiform movements are recorded separately.

ATHETOTIFORM MOVEMENTS (ATHETOID-LIKE MOVEMENTS; I-ATH)
These are small, slow movements, rather writhing in appearance, which occur quite irregularly and arrhythmically in different muscles. Presumably, they may occur in all muscles of the body, but are seen most easily in the muscles of the fingers and tongue.

In this test, the examiner should look for athetotiform movements in the fingers only. These are scored as follows:

> 0 = – no athetotiform movements visible, in particular none during arm extension;
> 1 = + 2–5 slow writhing movements during 20-second arm extension;
> 2 = ++ 6–10 writhing movements during 20-second arm extension;
> 3 = +++ continuous writhing movements during 20-second arm extension.

CHOREO–ATHETOTIC MOVEMENTS
These are usually associated with severe neurological diseases, but they are described here because of the difficulty of distinguishing them when they are of light intensity from less marked movements such as choreiform and athetotiform movements.

CHOREATIC MOVEMENTS (MOVEMENTS OF CHOREA)
These consist of rather gross, jerky movements occurring irregularly and arrhythmically in different muscles. The child may sometimes have difficulty in keeping his balance because of their amplitude and intensity. The bursts are longer and more gross in comparison with choreiform movements. Electromyographically, choreiform movements appear as short twitches, whereas choreatic movements appear as bursts of activity.

ATHETOID MOVEMENTS (ATHETOTIC MOVEMENTS)
These are slow, writhing movements, which occur continuously, irregularly, and arrhythmically in different muscles. They are usually of greater amplitude than athetotiform movements and often cause difficulty in balancing.

Athetotis and chorea are often present at the same time. In athetotic cerebral palsy resulting from kernicterus, athetotis is rarely present without chorea.

TREMOR (I-TR)
This consists of involuntary, rhythmical, alternating movements. A clear distinction must be made between a resting tremor and tremor that occurs during movement. In this test, the examiner should look for resting tremor only, in the fingers and forearms.

It is worth noting the frequency and regularity of the tremor. Fast and very regular oscillations of small amplitude are usually of minimal clinical significance, and may be caused by nervous tension. Rarely, such a tremor is based on a familial condition known as 'benign essential tremor'. When there is an association with (often slight) myoclonic jerks the rare diagnosis of paramyoclonus multiplex must be considered, and in this case the tremor is usually slightly more coarse. A non-essential tremor usually shows less regularity in its frequency and amplitude, particularly during movement.

This is scored as follows:

    0 = – no tremor present;
    1 = + barely discernible tremor;
    2 = ++ marked tremor of the fingers;
    3 = ++ marked tremor of the fingers and arms.

Significance
The presence of some athetotiform movements is common in children below 6 years of age, but these movements wane with increasing age. If they persist after the age of 5 years, they can be considered to be a sign of maturational delay of the nervous system.

The current prevalence of choreiform movements (scores 2 and 3) at school age is about 8%. After the onset of puberty choreiform movements are infrequently observed (Prechtl and Stemmer, 1962). In the 1950s and 1960s about 5% of children showed a marked form of choreiform movements (score 3; Prechtl and Stemmer, 1962); nowadays such marked choreiform dyskinesia is rare (personal observation). Choreiform movements are more common in boys than girls (Prechtl and Stemmer, 1962).

The specific significance of choreiform movements has been debated (Prechtl 1987; Shaffer et al, 1984). Rutter et al (1966) reported that choreiform movements were related to lower intelligence, but not to specific learning disorders or psychiatric disorders, whereas other studies have provided evidence that choreiform dyskinesia and specific learning problems and psychiatric disorders, such as hyperactivity and impulsivity, were associated (Prechtl and Stemmer, 1962; Lucas et al, 1965; Wolf and Hurwitz, 1966).

A slight tremor in children of school age may be related to the specifics of the testing situation (nervous tension). However, some types of tremor are of primary neurological origin (paresis, hereditary tremor, including the 'benign essential tremor') or of secondary neurological origin (thyrotoxicosis, intoxications). A parkinson-type is rarely found in children and its presence would clearly transgress the bounds of minor dysfunction.

Serious dyskinetic movement disorders such as chorea and athetosis are attributed to failure or dysfunction of the basal ganglia (Sanger and Mink, 2006). However, the precise pathophysiology and the exact contribution of the various parts of the basal ganglia to the different movement disorders are still unclear (Mink, 2003; Wolf and Singer, 2008).

Reaction to push against the shoulder during standing (Co)

Procedure (Figure 5.5)
The child is asked to stand upright with his head centred, his arms hanging freely and his feet about 5 cm apart. The examiner gives a gentle sideways push against the child's shoulder, the intensity of the push being graded according to the child's age and body proportions. By keeping her free hand on the contralateral side, at some distance from the child's body, the examiner can prevent the child with poor balance from falling. This gesture also reassures the child, and is especially important in young children. The child's ability to remain standing without a sideward placing of his contralateral leg is recorded.

Age
This test is suitable for all children of 4 years and over, if performed in a playful manner. In 4- and 5-year-olds an occasional sidestep may be used to keep balance.

Response
The child will try to preserve his balance by shifting his body to the ipsilateral side. If he does not succeed, he may bend to the contralateral side, show some abduction of the arms, and may eventually even sidestep to the contralateral side. Overshooting to the

Figure 5.5 Reaction to push against the shoulder during standing.

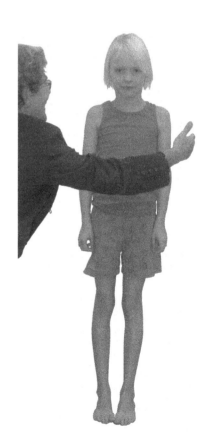

ipsilateral side may sometimes occur, and in this case, sidestepping may occur on that side.

Recording
Performance is scored as follows:

> 0 = typical response, keeps balance in an age-appropriate manner;
> 1 = mildly abnormal, uses sidestep too often for age;
> 2 = definitely abnormal, loses balance.

Consistent asymmetries, i.e. falling to one side, are recorded.

Significance
An inability to perform this test in an age-appropriate way may be caused by poor postural control because of muscle weakness (hypo- or hypertonia), postural abnormalities, or, most often, mild dysfunction in the supraspinal systems involved in postural control. Postural control is a task of reputed complexity in which virtually all parts of the nervous system are involved (Hadders-Algra and Brogren Carlberg, 2008).

Diadochokinesis (Co)

Procedure (Figure 5.6)
The child is required to stand with one arm relaxed at his side and the other flexed at an angle of about 90° at the elbow at about 10 cm distance from the body, the hand pointing forwards. The child's head must be centred and his arm and shoulder relaxed. Diadochokinesis consists of quickly pronating and supinating the hand and forearm. The examiner must demonstrate the movement at a speed of about three complete pronations and supinations per second. She then asks the child to imitate the movement. The child will start at his preferred speed and in his own way. He is allowed some practice trials. When the child extends the elbow during the movement, the examiner reminds the child to perform the movement with the elbow in flexion. Thereafter a new series of alternating pronations and supinations is started. When the child shows large abduction and adduction movements of the arm, reflected by large movements of the elbow, the examiner asks the child to try to keep the elbow as still as possible during the movement. When the child performs the movements slowly, the child is asked to move faster. Attention should be paid to the tendency to support the elbow against the body, as this may hide an inability to keep the elbow still.

Both arms are tested, but no specific order is requested. In general children start with their preferred arm.

Age
This test is applicable to children of 4 years and older. Performance improves with increasing age. Typical performance at 4 to 5 years consists of slow movements with

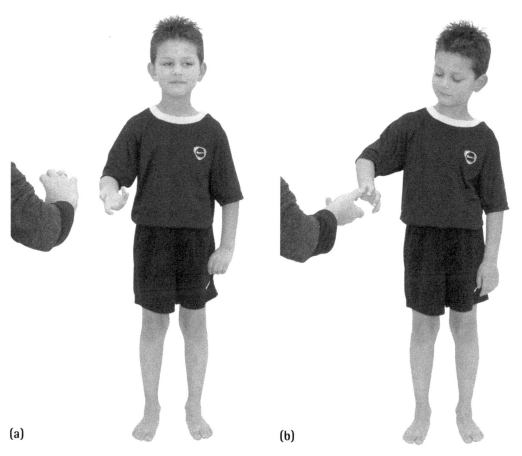

(a)   (b)

Figure 5.6 Diadochokinesis: (a) the arm is flexed at an angle of about 90° at the elbow at about a 10 cm distance from the body, the hand pointing forwards. Diadochokinesis consists of quickly pronating and supinating the hand and forearm. The contralateral arm hangs down relaxed. (b) Typical performance of a 7-year-old; this includes some elbow excursion and some associated activity in the contralateral arm.

large elbow excursions that usually show a minor pause at the extreme pronated and supinated positions of the hand (Table 5.1). By age 6 to 7 the test can be performed with more ease and at moderate speed (2–3 movement cycles per second), elbow excursion is limited to 5–15 cm, and conspicuous pauses at the extreme positions are no longer consistently present. In children aged 8 to 10 years elbow excursion is less than 5 cm. From 11 years onwards diadochokinesis can be performed quickly in a series of smoothly linked alternating pronation and supination movements with no or minor elbow movement.

AGE-RELATED CHANGES IN ASSOCIATED MOVEMENTS
Associated movements during diadochokinesis most often manifest themselves in the contralateral arm by associated pronation–supination movements. Other forms of

Table 5.1 Diadochokinesis: age-related changes in typical performance

	Age in years			
	4–5	6–7	8–10	>10
Elbow excursion (arm abduction and adduction)				
Mostly >15 cm	+	–	–	–
5–15 cm	–	+	–	–
<5 cm	–	–	+	+
Pauses at extreme positions of pronated and supinated hand				
Consistently	+	–	–	–
Occasionally	–	+	+	–
Absent	–	–	–	+
Speed				
Slow (1–2 cycles/s)	+	–	–	–
Moderate (2–3 cycles/s)	–	+	+	–
Fast (3–4 cycles/s)	–	–	–	+

+, typical performance for age (this does not exclude performance above average level for age); –, atypical for age.

associated activity are contralateral elbow flexion or to and fro sideward movements of the jaw.

Associated movement activity during diadochokinesis is characterized by large inter-individual variability. It may be more clearly expressed during performance of the non-dominant side, but the opposite may also occur. The degree of associated movements decreases with increasing age (Largo et al, 2001b). Marked associated movements in the contralateral arm may be seen in 4–6 year olds. Between 7 and 11 years typical performance is associated with some associated activity. From 12 years onwards diadochokinesis is performed with no or barely discernible associated activity.

Recording
This test is scored on two aspects: performance and associated movements. Each arm is assessed separately. Atypical performance is reflected by irregularity of movement and/or the absence of age-specific properties (Table 5.1).

(1) Performance is scored as follows:
    0 = typical, age-appropriate performance;
    1 = mildly abnormal: R, L, R & L;
    2 = definitely abnormal, serious difficulties in performance: R, L, R & L.

(2) Associated movements are scored as follows:

0 = absent;

1 = present, age-appropriate performance: R, L, R & L;

2 = present, exceeding age-appropriate norms: R, L, R & L.

Recording of associated movements: record what is happening during the performance on the side tested, e.g., R for associated activity occurring when the right hand performs diadochokinesis (and associated activity mainly is observed on the left side).

Significance
The test of diadochokinesis was developed by Joseph Babinski, the French neurologist whose name is connected to the pathological footsole reaction. Babinski noted that adults with a cerebellar lesion had difficulty in performing the test (Babinski, 1902). Later studies confirmed the finding of ipsilateral dysdiadochokinesis in patients with a cerebellar lesion (Wessel and Nitschke, 1997). More recently, the functional magnetic resonance imaging (MRI) studies of Tracy et al (2001) demonstrated marked activation of the ipsilateral cerebellum in healthy adults performing diadochokinesis. Yet, this study also revealed the substantial contribution to performance of other parts of the brain, such as the thalamus and the frontal and parietal cortices. The latter finding is in line with current concepts on the organization of motor control. Motor behaviour is considered to be continuously affected by distributed activity of cortical–subcortical circuitries organized in large-scale networks (Molinari et al, 2002). Notwithstanding the fact that diadochokinesis is the result of distributed brain activity, the contribution of the cerebellum is most important. This is illustrated by the finding that adults with an unilateral lesion caused by a cerebrovascular accident as a result of a stroke affecting one of the cerebral arteries, i.e. individuals with an intact cerebellum, are able to carry out diadochokinesis with an appropriate speed. Performance of individuals who have had a stroke is however characterized by reduced regularity of the alternating movement cycles, which underscores the notion of a non-cerebellar contribution to diadochokinesis (Hermsdörfer and Goldenberg, 2002).

Quite often an asymmetry between diadochokinesis on the two sides of the body may be observed. Such a discrepancy between the functioning of the right and left often increases with age, the pronation and supination improving at a faster rate on the dominant side. It is important to realize that mild asymmetries do not always correspond to side dominance. Marked asymmetries may be a sign of a hemisyndrome.

Interestingly, many children nowadays have difficulties in performing diadochokinesis, i.e. they show an irregular performance. In the 1980s and 1990s about 10% of school-age children exhibited such an irregular and inadequate performance, currently the prevalence has risen to 50% (personal observation). The background to this change over time is unknown, but it corresponds to other observations that children's motor abilities have deteriorated during the last few decades (Fleuren et al, 2007; Hadders-Algra, 2007). Based on the current high prevalence of inadequate performance on this test we changed the criterion for the domain of dysfunction 'coordination and balance' from 'more than one test inappropriate for age' to 'more than two tests inappropriate for age' (Hadders-Algra et al, 1988c, Peters et al, 2008).

Finger–nose test (Co)

Procedure (Figure 5.7)
The child is asked to put the tip of his index finger on the tip of his nose. The starting position consists of arm extension with an index finger ready to point (Figure 5.7a). The movements must be carried out relatively slowly and as accurately as possible. The test consists of a series of movements with the eyes open and movements with the eyes closed. Each series consists of three movements. The test starts with a series with the eyes open. A series using the same hand but with the eyes closed follows. Thereafter the other hand is tested, first with eyes open, then with eyes closed.

The examiner must demonstrate the test as she gives the instructions. Performance is facilitated, especially in the youngest children, when during the series with eyes open the examiner mirrors task performance. Some children persist in putting their finger on

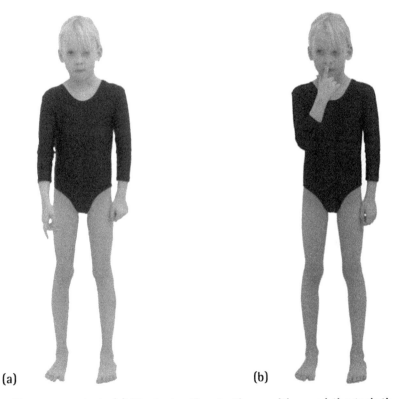

(a)   (b)

Figure 5.7 Finger–nose test: (a) illustrates the starting position and the task then consists of putting the tip of the index finger as accurately as possible on the tip of the nose (b).

the side of their nose or touching the bridge of the nose; in these cases, the examiner repeats the instruction that care should be taken to place the finger on the tip of the nose.

Age
If careful instructions are given this test can be performed from 4 years onwards.

Recording
The performance for each arm is assessed separately, and scored separately for the eyes open and the eyes closed condition. The assessment takes into account two aspects of performance: (1) smoothness of the movements and signs of intention tremor, and (2) success in placing the fingertip on the tip of the nose. Typically the finger follows a smooth trajectory through space before landing on the nose. Dysfunction may be reflected by the presence of a trajectory consisting of subunits of movements, i.e. minor halts in the movement during which the movement trajectory seems to be adjusted before continuing its path towards the nose. Dysfunction may also be reflected by the presence of an intention tremor. This tremor occurs at the end of a purposeful movement and may interfere with reaching the target in a pointing task. In addition, dysfunction may be expressed in the form of misplacement of the finger on e.g. the side of the nose.

Mild deviancy denotes the presence of a movement trajectory with clearly visible subunits, the presence of a slight tremor occurring only at the end of the movement, or one or two 'misses' of the nose. Marked deviancy implies the presence of a grossly abnormal movement trajectory, the presence of a marked intention tremor, or a consistent failure to touch the tip of the nose. Performance is scored as follows:

> 0 = typical, age-appropriate;
> 1 = mildly abnormal: R, L, R & L;
> 2 = definitely abnormal: R, L, R & L.

Consistent deviations or misplacings to one side should also be noted.

Significance
The Finger–nose test is a test of cerebellar function, although obviously sensory systems are also involved. In the eyes open situation the visual system and proprioception contribute; in the eyes closed situation only proprioception is involved.

The ability to produce a smooth movement towards the nose depends on the ability to programme the movement in advance (feedforward programming). The nervous system learns to produce predictive feedforward movements through trial and error. The learning process may be illustrated by the development of reaching. Reaching movements in early infancy are irregular and fragmented, they consist of multiple subunits of movement (Von Hofsten, 1991; Fallang et al, 2000). With increasing age and increasing experience including a multitude of self-produced trial and error situations, reaching movements become fluent, get a straight trajectory and, from 2 years onwards, consist of one or two movement subunits (Von Hofsten, 1991; Konczak and Dichgans, 1997; Kuhtz-Buschbeck et al, 1998). The cerebellum plays an important role in this type of trial and error learning. This is illustrated by the fact that cerebellar dysfunction may be reflected in movement trajectories that are not properly planned in advance and are characterized by an in-flight correction of movements based on peripheral feedback (Bastian, 2006).

Fingertip–touching test (Co)

Procedure (Figure 5.8)
The examiner stands or sits in front of the child and points an index finger at him, keeping her elbow flexed. The child is asked to put the tip of his index finger on the tip of the examiner's finger, the distance between them being such that the child has to flex his elbow to accomplish this. This also means that the tip of the examiner's finger is positioned at the level of the child's elbow.

Like the Finger–nose test, the Fingertip–touching test consists of a series of movements with eyes open and movements with eyes closed. Each series consists of three movements. The test starts with a series with eyes open. A series of the same hand with eyes closed follows. The latter task is difficult. The transition from the series with visual control to the series with eyes closed can be facilitated by the following procedure. When the child has placed his finger for the third time in the open eyes condition on the examiner's finger, the examiner holds the child's finger (with her contralateral hand) on the target finger. The child is told that he should continue with finger placements with the eyes closed meaning that he has to remember the feeling where his finger should go. When the child misses the target, the examiner places the child's finger on the target finger in order to provide the child with feedback on target location. After completion of the series with eyes closed the other hand is tested, first with eyes open, next with eyes closed. The examiner must take care not to change the position of her finger.

Age
The first part of the test is suitable for children older than 3 years as they are able to place their finger consistently on the tip of the target finger. The task with eyes closed can be performed from 5 years onwards. The number of correct placements in the absence of visual control increases with age (Table 5.2). But even adults frequently miss the target finger once.

Recording
Performance using each arm is assessed separately, and scored separately for the eyes open and the eyes closed condition. The assessment focuses on two aspects: (1) signs of intention tremor, and (2) success in placing the fingertip on the target finger.

A mild deviancy denotes the presence of a slight tremor occurring only at the end of the movement, or too many 'misses' of the target finger for age. Marked deviancy implies

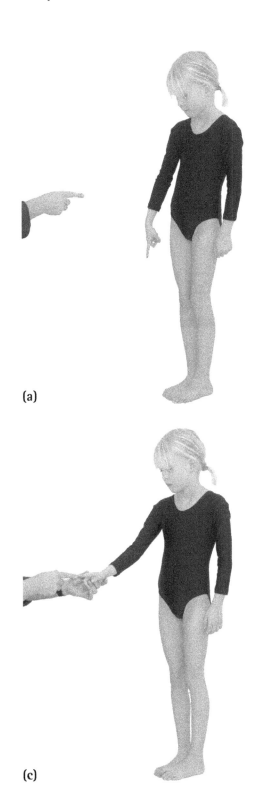

(a)

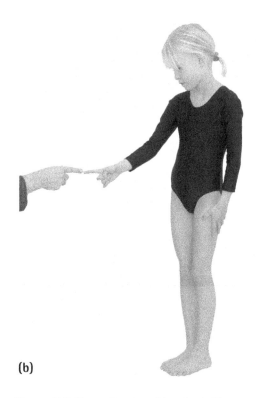

(b)

(c)

Figure 5.8 Fingertip–touching test: the child puts her finger on the tip of the examiner's finger. Note that the finger of the examiner is positioned so that the child can reach the tip of the examiner's finger by flexing the elbow 90°. (a) Starting position of the pointing finger, (b) end position of the pointing finger. (c) Before starting the series of pointing movements with eyes closed, the examiner holds the child's finger on the target finger while explaining that the finger target has to be remembered as the next trials should be performed with closed eyes.

Table 5.2 Fingertip–touching test: age-related changes in number of correct placements in the condition with eyes closed

Age, years	Number of correct placements	
	Dominant side	Non–dominant side
Below 5	0	0
5–6	1	0
6½–8	1	1
9–12	2	1
Over 12	2	2

the presence of a marked intention tremor in combination with a consistent failure to touch the target finger. Performance is scored as follows:

0 = typical, age-appropriate;

1 = mildly abnormal: R, L, R & L;

2 = definitely abnormal: R, L, R & L.

Consistent deviations or misplacings to one side should also be noted.

Significance
When the test is done with eyes open, visual guiding plays a preponderant role and, as such, the test gives some general information about hand–eye coordination. When carried out with eyes closed, cerebellar and proprioceptive systems are preponderant. The protracted developmental course of performance with eyes closed is presumably related to the developmental changes in the internal representations of the body in relation to the environment. At an early age children have a body-centred or egocentric reference frame (Rochat, 1998). At age 7–9 the egocentric reference frame, which mainly relies on somatosensory cues, is replaced by an exocentric reference frame, which is mainly based on gravitational cues (Contreras-Vidal et al, 2005; Roncesvalles et al, 2005).

Generally speaking, the presence of a tremor denotes cerebellar dysfunction, whereas deviations of placing reflect sensory proprioception dysfunction. Deviations that occur persistently to one side may be cerebellar or vestibular in origin.

Finger opposition test (F)

Procedure (Figure 5.9)
The examiner demonstrates to the child how to place the fingers of one hand (starting with the index finger) consecutively on the thumb of the same hand in the following sequence: 2, 3, 4, 5, 4, 3, 2, 3, 4, 5, etc. The child is asked to imitate these movements, completing five sequences to and fro (Figure 5.9a). The child is allowed some practise

(a)

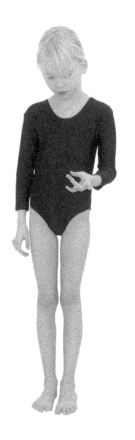

(b)

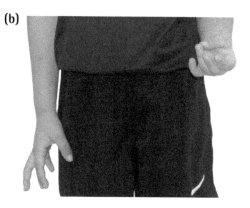

Figure 5.9 Finger opposition test: (a) placing the fingers (starting with the index finger) consecutively on the thumb in the following sequence: 2, 3, 4, 5, 4, 3, 2, 3, 4, 5, etc. (b) Note associated activity in the contralateral hand.

sequences. Each hand is tested in turn. The speed at which the test can be performed depends on the child's age. The elbow of the tested arm should not be pressed to the body. The contralateral arm hangs downwards relaxed.

Age
This test is applicable to children of 5 years and older. Some agile 4-year-olds are also able to perform it. Test performance shows large changes with increasing age (Table 5.3; Denckla, 1973, 1974; Largo et al, 2001a; Gasser et al, 2009).

Typical performance at 5 years consists of slow movements in one direction with many hesitations and many inappropriate movements of the other fingers of the same hand. By 6 years old children are able to change movement direction, but occasionally tap multiple times on the index finger or little finger before they change movement direction, reflecting difficulties in finger-to-finger transition. Performance is slow, with hesitations and many inappropriate movements of the other fingers of the same hand. Finger-to-finger transition in children aged 7–9 years resembles that of 6-year-olds but smoothness is better at this age: the test can be performed at moderate speed with less inappropriate movements of the other fingers. Movement transition becomes prompt and adequate at 10 years of age. Smoothness of movements in children aged 10–11 is similar to that in children aged 7–9 years. Smoothness is optimal for the first time at 13 years of age.

Table 5.3 Age-related changes in typical performance on the finger opposition test

	Age in years						
	4	5	6	7–9	10–11	12	≥13
Appropriate sequence (T)^a							
In one direction	–	+	–	–	–	–	–
In both directions	–	–	+	+	+	+	+
Change in movement direction (T)^b							
Taps usually >1×	–	+	–	–	–	–	–
Taps occasionally >1×	–	–	+	+	–	–	–
Prompt switch	–	–	–	–	+	+	+
Movements of inappropriate fingers (not touching thumb) (S)^c							
Marked movements	–	+	+	–	–	–	–
Minor movements	–	–	–	+	+	–	–
No movements	–	–	–	–	–	+	+
Smoothness of movement (S)^d							
With large hesitation	–	+	–	–	–	–	–
With some hesitation	–	–	+	+	+	+	–
No hesitation, smooth	–	–	–	–	–	–	+
Speed of performance (S)^e							
Slow	–	+	+	–	–	–	–
Moderate	–	–	–	+	+	–	–
Quick	–	–	–	–	–	+	+

S, relating to the smoothness of movement; T, relating to the criterion of finger-to-finger transition; +, typical performance for age (this does not exclude performance above average level for age); –, atypical for age.

a. Appropriate sequence: child is able to produce a movement sequence in one direction (2, 3, 4, 5 or 5, 4, 3, 2) or in both directions irrespective of the adequacy of change in movement direction.

b. Change in movement direction: the number of taps the child produces on index finger or little finger when changing movement direction.

c. Movements of inappropriate fingers: movements of fingers-not-in-turn-to-tap on the same hand.

d. Smoothness of movement: the degree of hesitation of the tapping finger to touch the thumb; also very large movements of the tapping fingers are regarded as non-smooth movements.

e. Speed of performance: slow, 1–2 taps/second; moderate, 2–3 taps/second; quick, 3–4 taps/second.

Performance of the test is improved by practising and thus by laterality, i.e. in general the dominant hand performs slightly better than the non-dominant hand. Skilled finger opposition develops in general somewhat faster in girls than in boys (Denckla, 1974; Largo et al, 2001a; Gasser et al, 2009).

AGE-RELATED CHANGES IN ASSOCIATED MOVEMENTS
Associated movements during the finger opposition test consist of finger movements of the contralateral hand (Figure 5.9b). The degree of associated movements decreases with increasing age (Largo et al, 2001b; Gasser et al, 2009). Children of 5 and 6 show marked associated movements in the contralateral hand. In children aged 7 to 9 usually some associated activity can be observed in the contralateral hand. Children of 10 years and over show no or a minimal amount of associated movements in the other hand.

Recording
This test is scored on three aspects of performance and each arm is assessed separately.

(1) Finger-to-finger transition i.e. the transition from one finger to the next in the right order, especially at the turning points involving the index and the little fingers. This is scored as follows:

    0 = typical, age-appropriate performance;

    1 = mildly abnormal: R, L, R & L;

    2 = definitely abnormal, serious difficulties in performance: R, L, R & L.

(2) Smoothness of movement, governed by movements of other fingers of the same hand, hesitations in placing the correct finger and the speed of performance. This is scored as follows:

    0 = typical, age-appropriate performance;

    1 = mildly abnormal: R, L, R & L;

    2 = definitely abnormal, serious difficulties in performance: R, L, R & L.

(3) Associated movements in the opposite hand. This is scored as follows:

    0 = absent;

    1 = present, age-appropriate performance: R, L, R & L;

    2 = present, exceeding age-appropriate norms: R, L, R & L.

Significance
The finger opposition test belongs to the domain of fine manipulation. This complex motor task consists of self-initiated sequential finger movements. Functional imaging studies demonstrated that self-initiated sequential finger movements in adults are associated with widespread cortical activity in frontal and parietal areas, including bilateral activity in the primary motor and primary sensory cortex, premotor areas, the supplementary motor area, and the limbic cingulate cortex (Gordon et al, 1998; Wu and Hallett, 2005; Mostofsky et al, 2006). The activity in the primary motor cortex and, to a lesser extent, in the primary sensory cortex is larger on the contralateral than on the ipsilateral side; a similar contralateral dominance is not present in the other cortical areas

(Baraldi et al, 1999). Self-initiated sequential finger movements are not only associated with cortical activity, but also with increased activity in the basal ganglia (contralaterally more than ipsilaterally), midbrain (e.g. substantia nigra), and cerebellum (ipsilaterally more than contralaterally; Wu and Hallett, 2005; Boecker et al, 2008).

Follow-a-finger test (F)

Procedure (Figure 5.10 and 5.11)
The child is asked to keep the tip of his index finger at a distance of 0.5–1 cm from the examiner's index finger, and to follow the examiner's movements closely. The examiner's hand describes a pattern in various vertical and horizontal directions, with some angles of 90° (Figure 5.11). Both hands are tested consecutively.

Age
The performance on the follow-a-finger test depends on the child's age (Table 5.4). Children of 4 and 5 years have difficulties in performing the test. They jerkily follow the

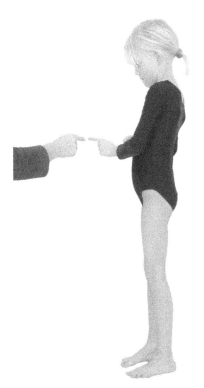

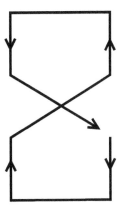

Figure 5.10 Starting position for the follow-a-finger test: in front of the child's body with a small gap between the examiner's and the child's finger.

Figure 5.11 Schematic drawing of movement sequences during follow-a-finger test.

examiner's finger with considerable delay and produce large gaps between the leading finger of the examiner and their own finger. Performance is better in children of 6 years and over; they perform the test without gross jerks or tremors. With increasing age the gap between the fingers of the examiner and the child at the change in movement direction becomes smaller to reach the minimum value of less than 2 cm at the age of 11 years. At 10 years the movement becomes less jerky. It is important to appreciate that the following movement, in general, is not performed with perfect smoothness. At school age the movement is carried out at moderate speed; from 12 years onwards the

Table 5.4 Follow-a-finger test: age-related changes in typical performance

	Age in years					
	4–5	6	7–9	10	11	≥13
Delay in change of movement direction						
Considerable delay	+	−	−	−	−	−
Follows relatively prompt	−	+	+	+	+	+
Gap^a at change in movement direction						
10–20 cm	+	−	−	−	−	−
Usually ±5 cm, but occasionally ±10 cm	−	+	−	−	−	−
<5 cm	−	−	+	−	−	−
Usually ±2 cm, but occasionally ±5 cm	−	−	−	+	−	−
<2 cm	−	−	−	−	+	+
Fluency of movement^b						
Jerky	+	+	+	−	−	−
Somewhat non-fluent	−	−	−	+	+	+
Fluent	−	−	−	−	−	−
Speed of performance^c						
Slow	+	−	−	−	−	−
Moderate	−	+	+	+	+	−
Quick	−	−	−	−	−	+

+, typical performance for age (this does not exclude performance above average level for age); −, atypical for age.

a. Gap between finger of examiner and finger of child at turning point, i.e. overshoot or undershoot.

b. Fluency of movement: jerky, frequent presence of jerky movements; somewhat non-fluent, presence of minor degree of non-fluency, no overt jerks, tremor, or stiffness.

c. Speed: slow, 10–15 cm/second; moderate, 5–10 cm/second; quick, 2–5 cm/second.

child is able to follow quickly. In general performance of the dominant hand is slightly better than that of the non-dominant hand.

Recording
Attention is paid to any overshooting or undershooting during changes in the direction of movement, to the smoothness of movement and to the speed with which the movement can be performed. Each arm is assessed separately as follows:

0 = normal, age-appropriate performance;
1 = mildly abnormal: R, L, R & L;
2 = definitely abnormal, serious difficulties in performance: R, L, R & L.

Significance
The follow-a-finger test belongs to the domain of fine manipulation. It is a complex motor task involving widespread cortical activity including activity of the frontal (primary motor, premotor, and supplementary motor cortex), parietal, and occipital cortex and activity of the cerebellum (Lacquaniti et al, 1997; Miall et al, 2001; Goodale and Westwood, 2004).

Circle test (F)

Procedure (Figure 5.12 and 5.13)
The first series of circles consists of large circles. The examiner draws circles in the air with her arms extended at the elbows during the parts of the circles at which the hands move away from the body. She makes the movements with both arms simultaneously but in opposite directions. The child is asked to copy the movements. After completing five circles (the examiner counts aloud), the movement is repeated in the reverse direction with a series of five circles. Then, without a pause, the circular movements are made with both arms in the same direction. After completion of five circles in this way, the direction is reversed, again with a series of five circles. The second series consists of small circles. The examiner draws circles in the air with her extended index finger, wrist and forearm (elbow semi-flexed); the elbows should be kept still during the small circles. The child is asked to copy again two series of five circles in the opposite direction (turning outwards, turning inwards) and two series of five circles in the same direction (clockwise and counter clockwise). Care should be taken that the child does not press the elbows to the body and that the hands do not touch each other but perform the movements individually.

Age
Four-year-olds are only able to produce oval shaped large circles in the opposite direction.

Children aged 5 years can perform circular movements in the opposite and same direction, usually with some hesitation at the change in movement direction. Large circles in the opposite direction are performed in a coordinated way with a mix of oval

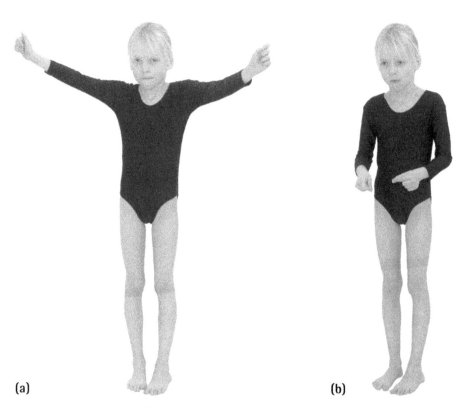

(a) (b)

Figure 5.12 Circle test: (a) large circles, involving in particular movements in the shoulder joints; elbows more or less extended, (b) small circles, involving in particular movements in the elbow joints; elbows more or less flexed.

and round circles, small circles in the opposite direction are performed with less coordination and are not round. Five-year-olds can produce large, coordinated and oval shaped movements in the same direction. They cannot produce small circles in the same direction.

Performance in producing the circles gradually improves with increasing age (Table 5.5). Development of circles in the opposite direction precedes that of the circles in the same direction. Large and small circles in the opposite direction can be performed in a synchronous and coordinated way from 6 years onwards. Large circles in the opposite direction have a round form at 7 years, the small circles in the opposite direction are performed in a consistently round form from 11 years onwards.

Movement coordination of circles in the same direction develops considerably slower. An appropriate coordination of movements during large and small movements occurs first in children aged 13 years and over. The transition from one movement pattern (series of circles) to another movement pattern is prompt in children of 7 years and over.

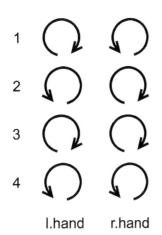

Figure 5.13 Schematic drawing of movement sequences in the circle test.

l.hand   r.hand

Recording
Attention is paid to movement synchrony, pattern coordination, the form of the circles, and the child's ability to make the transition from one movement pattern to another movement pattern.

(1) Opposite direction is scored as follows:
    0 = typical, age-appropriate performance;
    1 = mildly abnormal: R, L, R & L;
    2 = definitely abnormal, serious difficulties in performance: R, L, R & L.
(2) Same direction is scored as follows:
    0 = typical, age-appropriate performance;
    1 = mildly abnormal: R, L, R & L;
    2 = definitely abnormal, serious difficulties in performance: R, L, R & L.
(3) Transition is scored as follows:
    0 = immediately follows changes of direction;
    1 = has problems in the transition from one movement form into another.

Significance
The circle test belongs to the domain of fine manipulation. The bimanual circle task during which hands cycle in the opposite direction involves a symmetric mode of movement coordination and the task during which the hands move in the same direction an asymmetric mode. The symmetric mode requires less neuronal computation than the asymmetric one as the latter task requires recruitment of non-homologous muscles (Carson et al, 1997).

The circle test, in particular, evaluates cooperation between the right and left frontal and parietal cortices, in which is the corpus callosum plays a prominent role (Stanćák et al, 2003; Fryer et al, 2008). Indeed, patients who have undergone resection of the corpus

Table 5.5 Circle test: age-related changes in typical performance

	Age in years						
	4	5	6	7–9	10–11	12	≥13
Opposite direction							
Movement synchrony							
During large circles only	+	–	–	–	–	–	–
During large and small circles	–	+	+	+	+	+	+
Pattern coordination[a]							
During large circles only	+	+	–	–	–	–	–
During large and small circles	–	–	+	+	+	+	+
Form of large circles							
Oval forms	+	–	–	–	–	–	–
Mix of oval and round forms	–	+	+	–	–	–	–
Round forms	–	–	–	+	+	+	+
Form of small circles							
Oval forms	–	+	–	–	–	–	–
Mix of oval and round forms	–	–	+	+	+	–	–
Round forms	–	–	–	–	–	+	+
Same direction							
Movement synchrony[b]							
During large circles only	–	+	–	–	–	–	–
During large and small circles	–	–	+	+	+	+	+
Pattern coordination[a]							
During last large circles only	–	+	+	–	–	–	–
During most large circles	–	–	–	+	+	–	–
During all large and most small circles	–	–	–	–	–	+	–
During large and small circles	–	–	–	–	–	–	+
Form of large circles							
Oval forms	–	+	–	–	–	–	–
Mix of oval and round forms	–	–	+	+	+	–	–
Round forms	–	–	–	–	–	+	+
Form of small circles							
Oval forms	–	–	+	–	–	–	–
Mix of oval and round forms	–	–	–	+	+	+	–
Round forms	–	–	–	–	–	–	+
Transition							
After a few attempts	–	+	+	–	–	–	–
Promptly	–	–	–	+	+	+	+

callosum for intractable epilepsy show difficulties in spatial and temporal coupling of bimanual movements (Eliassen et al, 1999; Kennerley et al, 2002).

The extended period over which improvements in an individual's performance on the circle test occurs matches the protracted development of the frontal and parietal cortices and corpus callosum. The development of these structures extends into adolescence with an interesting transition around 12 years of age: the volumes of frontal and parietal grey matter reach their peak and callosal function allows, for the first time, the interhemispheric achievement of a bimanual procedural task (De Guise and Lassonde, 2001; Lenroot and Giedd, 2006).

Notes for Table 5.5 (opposite)

+, typical performance for age; this does not exclude performance above average level for age;
−, a typical for age.

a. Pattern coordination reflects the spatial coupling of the movements of both arms, i.e. the degree to which movement trajectories of both arms are coordinated.

b. Movement synchrony reflects the temporal coupling of the movements of both arms: both arms move at similar rhythm and speed.

Chapter 6

Assessment of the child walking

Ability to walk

The ability to walk with or without help is recorded. The inability to walk without support indicates the presence of major neurological dysfunction or other serious pathology. The presence of minor neurological dysfunction (MND) does not interfere with the ability to walk without support.

Posture during walking (PT)

Procedure
The child walks up and down the assessment room (or corridor) a few times. To avoid increased self-awareness of walking behaviour, which may induce an unnatural way of walking, the child may be given the task of going to fetch an object from the other side of the room.

Age
Walking can be evaluated from early childhood onwards.

Recording
The following aspects of walking behaviour are assessed:

(1) posture during walking;
(2) gait width;
(3) heel–toe gait; and
(4) quality of gait.

POSTURE DURING WALKING
Posture of head, trunk, arms, legs, and feet is scored separately as follows:

> 0 = typical;
> 1 = mildly abnormal;
> 2 = definitely abnormal.

Special attention should be paid to movements of the arms and movements of the hip and knees. If flexion of the hip, knee and/or ankle is impaired on one side, the child will compensate for this by circumducting the leg in an arc away from the hip. In extreme cases, such as spastic hemiplegia with equinovarus posture of the foot, the pelvis will be raised on the affected side and the toes may still scrape against the floor.

The position of the feet in relation to the lower leg is noted, with special attention being paid to possible valgus postures causing the child to walk on the instep of the foot. Asymmetries or other deviations of posture resulting, for instance, from slight scoliosis, slight diffuse hypotonia or asymmetrical, mainly static, foot posture, which are present when the child is standing, may disappear during walking. The reverse may also happen. The phenomena should be described.

GAIT WIDTH
The distance between the feet is 10–20 cm in children over 2½–3 years during typical gait (Hempel, 1993a and 1993b). Gait is scored as follows:

> 0 = typical;
> 1 = abnormal: narrow/broad;

HEEL–TOE GAIT
In normal gait the heel touches the ground first and the weight of the body is then shifted to the toes with an arching of the foot. This pattern, which is established during the second year (Cioni et al, 1993), is referred to as the 'heel–toe' gait. This is scored as follows:

> 0 = appropriate heel–toe gait;
> 1 = mildly abnormal: does not appropriately roll from heel to toe or walks occasionally on tiptoes.
> 2 = walks consistently on tiptoes.

QUALITY OF GAIT
This is scored as follows:

> 0 = typical;
> 1 = abnormal, e.g. remarkably jerky, sloppy, or stiff.

Significance

Asymmetries in the posture of the head or trunk during walking may be the result of neurological or orthopaedic causes (e.g. hemiplegia or rheumatoid arthritis). In cases of generalized hypotonia, the posture may be symmetrical but abnormal. Asymmetries in arm or leg movements may be signs of mild lateralization or hemisyndrome.

Children below the age of 6 quite often show only minimal arching of the foot, in extreme cases the foot may even be exorotated and pronated (walking on the instep). Often these children cannot walk long distances and tire easily on walking trips. Generally, no arching of the foot is visible when the child is standing still. A perpendicular line from the internal malleolus reaching the floor outside the circumference of the footprint indicates talipes valgus. At this age, this is usually the result of lax ligaments around the ankle joints, and postural deviations generally disappear during the course of the next few years as the ligaments grow stronger. There may be a neurological cause such as hypotonia, but this is rare. Most so-called 'flatfeet' at this age are really talipes valgus disorders. Treatment with arch supports (which do not affect the underlying cause) are of little value: the ideal treatment is the introduction of strong shoes that support the ankle joints and counteract the tendency to walk on the instep. Asymmetries and extreme cases of symmetrical talipes valgus must be carefully examined as they may be of neurological origin (e.g. lateralization, hypotonia, isolated hypertonia).

Children below the age of 5 tend to show only a few arm movements while walking, the 4-year-old generally keeping his arms still.

In children over the age of 6, arching of the foot should be evident during walking and should generally be visible during standing flat and on tiptoes. If the posture of the ankle joint is adequate but there is no arching, pes planus should be suspected. Static or hereditary factors are important in most cases. In cases of marked pes planus, a symmetrical abduction posture of the feet is usual.

Walking on the instep is usually a sign of mild hypotonia in children over the age of 6 or 7, but it can also be an early sign of progressive muscle weakness.

Circumduction of one leg results from inadequate integration of knee and/or ankle movements in locomotion, and may be a result of nervous dysfunction (such as spastic hemiparesis) or arthrogenic, or myogenic causes. In cases of mild hypertonia on one side of the body, circumduction may be evident before the examination of the resistance against passive movements reveals any difference between the two legs. This must be differentiated from the effects of pain, which, by immobilizing joints, may also lead to some degree of circumduction.

In normal gait, the distance between the feet remains constant. A variable width of gait may be arthrogenic (e.g. luxation or subluxation of the hip joint) or neurological in origin, although once again this must be differentiated from a variable width of gait because of pain. A very narrow gait may result from hypertonia of the adductor muscles of the leg, which, in cases of mild diplegia, can occur without any evidence of scissoring of the legs. A wide gait may be caused by nervous dysfunction (e.g. muscular hypotonia of the leg and/or pelvic girdle, sensory, or cerebellar dysfunction) or may be arthrogenic in origin, as in the case of luxation or subluxation of the hip joint.

Dipping and strong swinging movements of the hips may be caused by muscle diseases (e.g. gluteal muscle weakness) or by hip dysplasia, the latter sometimes resulting from hypertonia (e.g. spasticity of internal pelvic rotatory muscles and/or leg adductors). However, swinging movements of the hips during walking can also occur in cases of hypotonia and in cases of hypertonia without hip dysplasia. Obviously, hip subluxations independent of neurological disease will lead to distorted hip movements during walking, with a marked dipping of the pelvis with each stride. Children who are accustomed to sitting on the floor between flexed legs may show a gait characterized by a moderate amount of swinging movements of the hips and changing width of gait. This is caused by a lengthening of the abductors and a shortening of the adductors of the upper leg as a result of the posture when sitting. This posture is chosen by children who are slightly hypotonic.

Consistently walking on tiptoe may be the expression of a neurodevelopmental disorder such as spastic cerebral palsy, muscular dystrophy, or autism (Gardner-Medwin and Johnston, 1984; Farmer, 2003; Ming et al, 2007). Walking on tiptoe may also occur as an isolated dysfunction. The aetiology of this idiopathic toe walking is largely unknown, but it may have a genetic origin (Sala et al, 1999). In most children with idiopathic toe walking their walking has normalized in adolescence or adulthood (Hirsch and Wagner, 2004).

It must be borne in mind that the individual's foot postures can vary considerably during walking, and that findings may therefore be rather difficult to interpret. Marked exo- or endorotation or marked dorsi- or plantar flexion should arouse suspicion of an abnormality, as should any obvious asymmetries. However, as with other signs, a final interpretation can only be made when a full examination has been completed.

Abnormalities in the quality of gait may be an unspecific indicator of neural dysfunction.

Walking along a straight line (Co)

Procedure (Figure 6.1)
The child is asked to walk along a straight line for approximately 20 continuous paces and then back again. One foot should be placed directly in front of the other. No specific instructions about arm behaviour are given.

Age
The test can be carried out from 4 year onwards. However, 4-year-olds in general need some space between the feet and an occasional sidestep to cover task trajectory. Five-year-olds can perform the steps without distance between the feet and without sidesteps. Stepping behaviour at this age is usually characterized by irregularity in stepping and the

Figure 6.1 Walking along a straight line: one foot should be placed directly in front of the other.

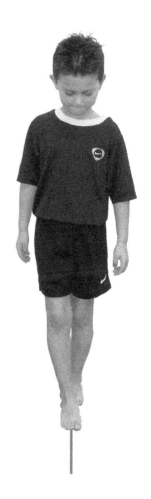

presence of large arm movements. From 6 years onwards, stepping behaviour is more regular and arm movements are used to a limited extent only. From 9 years onwards stepping is performed regularly without balancing movements of the arms.

Recording
Performance should be scored as follows:

0 = typical, age-appropriate;
1 = mildly abnormal;
2 = definitely abnormal, cannot perform or frequently loses balance.

Consistent asymmetries, i.e. falling to one side, are recorded.

Significance
Walking along a line is primarily a test of balance and body coordination. Poor performance may be a result of hypotonia, hypertonia, cerebellar, or sensory

dysfunction. Moreover, involuntary movements such as choreiform dyskinesia or tremor (high intensity) may interfere with the child's performance. Persisting deviations to one side may reflect a hemisyndrome of cerebellar or non-cerebellar origin.

Walking on tiptoe

Procedure (Figure 6.2)
The child is asked to walk on tiptoe for approximately 20 paces and then back again.

Age
Children over 3 years of age should be able to walk on tiptoe.

AGE-RELATED CHANGES IN ASSOCIATED MOVEMENTS
Associated movement activity while walking on toes is characterized by large inter-individual variability. Four-year-olds in general show marked associated activity in the form of arm, wrist and finger extension, and facial activity, including tongue movements. From 5 years onwards associated activity is restricted to some extension of the wrist and fingers. After the onset of puberty associated activity is virtually absent (Largo et al, 2001b).

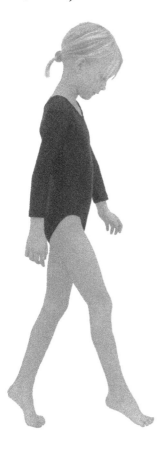

Figure 6.2 A 7-year-old girl demonstrates: walking on toes with only minimal associated activity in the arms (in the left arm in the form of some elbow extension and some dorsiflexion of the wrist).

Recording
This test is scored on two aspects: performance and associated movements.

(1) Walking on tiptoe is scored as follows:
> 0 = typical, age-appropriate performance;
> 1 = mildly abnormal, difficulties in performance: R, L, R & L;
> 2 = definitely abnormal, cannot perform: R, L, R & L.

(2) Associated movements (A) are scored as follows:
> 0 = absent;
> 1 = present, age-appropriate performance: R, L, R & L;
> 2 = present, exceeding age-appropriate norms: R, L, R & L.

Significance
A poor performance may be as a result of hypotonia or flexor hypertonia, and a very good performance may be because of extensor hypertonia. Asymmetries may indicate a lateralization syndrome and should be carefully investigated after having first established that there are no deformities of the feet or other possible non-neurological causes. Individuals with mild hemisyndromes may present with walking on tiptoe and on heels before they can be seen in ordinary walking or can be felt while testing the resistance against passive and active movements. Corroboration of the unilateral findings can usually then be obtained by inspecting the sitting posture, standing posture, and the posture of the legs and feet while the child is lying in prone and supine positions. Bilateral foot deformities may also influence performance.

Walking on heels

Procedure (Figure 6.3)
The child is asked to walk on his heels over a distance of approximately 20 paces and then back again.

Age
Children over the age of 3 years should be able to walk on their heels.

AGE-RELATED CHANGES IN ASSOCIATED MOVEMENTS
Associated movement activity while walking on heels is characterized by large inter-individual variability. In general 4- and 5-year-olds show marked associated activity in the form of some shoulder abduction, marked elbow flexion in combination with hyperextension of the wrists, and marked associated activity in the face and tongue. The degree of associated activity decreases gradually with increasing age (Largo et al, 2001b). In general, children aged 6 or 7 years show some shoulder abduction, elbow flexion not exceeding 90°, wrist hyperextension, and some facial activity. From 8 years onwards associated activity is reduced to minor degrees of elbow flexion and some wrist hyperextension. Associated activity may disappear after the onset of puberty, but this is not always the case (Largo et al, 2001b).

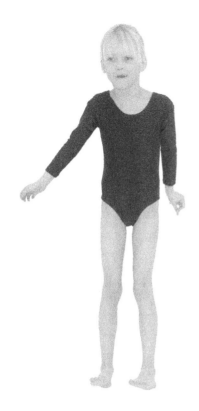

Figure 6.3 A 7-year-old girl demonstrates: walking on heels with associated activity in the face and arms.

The finding that associated activity during walking on heels is more intensive and persists longer during development than associated activity during walking on toes reflects the difference in the difficulty of the two tasks (Wolff et al, 1983). Associated activity can be observed in particular during difficult and complex tasks (Largo et al, 2001b).

Recording
This test is scored on two aspects: performance and associated movements. Appropriate performance means that the child is able to walk at least 15 paces on heels, i.e. with forefoot, including lateral parts of the forefoot, lifted off the floor.

(1) Walking on heels is scored as follows:

0 = typical, age-appropriate performance;

1 = mildly abnormal, difficulties in performance: R, L, R & L;

2 = definitely abnormal, cannot perform: R, L, R & L.

(2) Associated movements (A) are scored as follows:

0 = absent;

1 = present, age-appropriate performance: R, L, R & L;

2 = present, exceeding age-appropriate norms: R, L, R & L.

Significance

Classically a poor performance has been associated with hypotonia of the lower leg muscles or paresis. It is of particular interest to note here that paresis of the peroneal muscles may occur without other muscles being impaired to the same degree. The child will walk on the outer side of the foot rather than on the heels, or, in mild cases, will commence walking on the heel but will fail and soon afterwards will walk on endorotated feet. Children with mild hypotonia who walked on the instep during the test for ordinary walking may show the same phenomenon, with no signs of muscle paresis. Children without hypotonia who walk on the instep (mainly children under 6 years of age) usually walk normally on the heels. As already stated in the section on walking on tiptoe, the presence of a mild hemisyndrome may be discovered by close inspection of the symmetry of walking on heels. Clearly, any foot deformities will interfere with performance. Asymmetries may indicate a lateralization syndrome or they may result from non-neurological causes (e.g. unilateral foot deformities, arthogenic origins).

Poor performance during walking on heels is however more closely associated with fine manipulative disability and coordination problems than with mild dysregulation of muscle tone (personal observation). The association with problems with fine manipulation and coordination problems may reflect the relatively large contribution of supraspinal control to ankle dorsiflexors that is involved in walking on heels. Supraspinal control of ankle dorsiflexors is considerably larger than that of ankle plantar flexors; which are used during walking on tiptoe (Dietz 1992, Hadders-Algra 1998). The suggestion that the ability to walk on heels is related to the integrity of supraspinal integrity is supported by the findings of Olsén et al (1997) that poor performance in walking on heels is associated with abnormalities in the periventricular white matter.

Standing on one leg (Co)

Procedure (Figure 6.4)

The child is asked to stand on one leg as long as possible. The examiner counts the seconds out loud. When the child has performed the task for 20 seconds the examiner tells the child that the task has been accomplished. When the child ends the task before 20 seconds have elapsed, one or two other trials are performed. The best result is recorded. Each leg is tested in turn, the child being allowed to start with whichever leg he prefers.

Age

The ability to stand on one leg develops quite suddenly and improves rapidly (Sutherland et al, 1988). The minimum criteria for typical development are as follows: at 4 years the child should be able to stand on the preferred leg for at least 3 seconds; around the fifth birthday this has improved to 5 seconds; at 5½ years children should be able to carry on for 10 and 13 seconds (non-preferred and preferred leg, respectively); at 6, this has improved to 13 and 16 seconds; and by the age of 7, children should be able to stand on one leg for more than 20 seconds. Initially children use all parts of the body

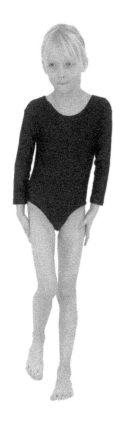

Figure 6.4 Standing on one leg. No instructions are given about how to position the arms and legs.

to maintain balance; these balancing movements disappear with increasing age. In children over 10 toe flexion and swaying movements of the body and arms should be absent.

Recording
The performance of each leg is recorded in terms of the duration of achievement in seconds and the quality of motor behaviour, i.e. the presence of toe flexion (yes/no) and swaying movements of body and arms (yes/no). Performance is scored as follows:

   0 = typical, age-appropriate;
   1 = mildly abnormal;
   2 = definitely abnormal, serious difficulties in performance.

Mildly abnormal performance indicates that the child is able to perform the task to some extent, but not in an age-appropriate manner. This means in the youngest age groups that the duration of standing on one leg is too short for age, in children older than 10 it may also mean the presence of toe flexion and swaying movements. The score 'definitely abnormal' can only be applied from 7 years onwards, i.e. from the age at which a 20-second performance typically has been achieved. Definitely abnormal means that a child is unable to stand on one leg for longer than 1 or 2 seconds.

Significance
Standing on one leg is a test that evaluates static balance and body coordination. Its protracted developmental course reflects the complex nature of the postural control mechanisms involved (Hadders-Algra and Brogren Carlberg, 2008).

Poor performance is especially related to coordination problems. It may also be associated with deviancies in the regulation of muscle tone and the presence of involuntary movements. For instance the sudden jerks of proximal choreiform movements may nearly throw the child off balance, thereby interfering with performance.

Typically, achievement on one leg is better than on the other. This means that asymmetries should be interpreted with caution. Extreme cases of asymmetry may reflect a lateralization syndrome, in which case there will undoubtedly be other signs of nervous dysfunction, which show an analogous pattern.

Hopping (Co)

Procedure
The child is asked to hop on each foot at least 20 times, starting with whichever leg he prefers. Hopping on the spot is best, but children younger than 9 years often cannot manage this and so should be allowed to move forwards. The child is asked to hop on his toes, and not with the whole foot. Hopping on the whole foot can be heard as well as seen.

Age
The development of this motor function is abrupt and rapid. The minimum criteria for typical development are as follows: at 4 years children should be able to hop three times on one foot (not on the other). At 5 years 3 and 5 hops should be achieved (non-preferred and preferred leg, respectively), at 5½ to 6 years 10 and 13 hops respectively, whereas from 6½ to 7 years onwards 20 hops should be performed on each leg. Further refinement of hopping behaviour consists of the ability to hop on the spot from 9 years onwards and the ability to hop consistently on toes. The latter is however first achieved in all children after the onset of puberty; in 10- to 12-year-olds 60–80% of children are able to hop on their toes.

Recording
The performance of each foot is recorded separately. The number of hops, with a maximum of 20, is recorded and whether the child is able to hop on the spot (yes/no) and on toes (yes/no). Performance is scored as follows:

    0 = typical, age-appropriate;

    1 = mildly abnormal;

    2 = definitely abnormal, serious difficulties in performance.

Mildly abnormal performance indicates that the child is able to perform the task to some extent, but not in an age-appropriate manner. This means in the youngest age groups that too few hops for age are produced, in children of 9 years and over it may also imply the inability to hop on the spot. The score 'definitely abnormal performance' can only be applied from 7 years onwards, i.e. from the age at which typical performance consists of 20 hops. Definitely abnormal means that a child is unable to produce more than two hops.

Significance
Hopping is a test that evaluates dynamic balance and body coordination (Roberton and Halverson, 1988). Poor hopping may reflect the presence of coordination problems and dysfunctional muscle tone regulation. Interestingly, children with the latter type of dysfunctions more often exhibit problems in standing on one leg than in the dynamic test of hopping. Hopping on the whole foot in older children usually reflects hypotonia.

Mild asymmetries in performance are part and parcel of typical development. This means that an asymmetrical performance must be very carefully interpreted. The greater the discrepancy between left and right, the greater the possibility of a hemisyndrome or other lateralization syndrome as the underlying cause. If such a lateralization is present, other neurological findings should corroborate it.

Chapter 7

Assessment of the child lying

The child is asked to lie on his back with his arms by his sides, either on the floor or on a mattress on the floor. In this position the knee–heel test is performed (see below). After completion of the knee–heel test the child is asked to stand up.

The examiner observes the quality of posture and motility during the lying down and standing up procedures. During standing up special attention is paid to the presence of Gower's sign, i.e. the 'climbing up the legs' that indicates weakness of truncal and proximal lower extremity muscles. Gower's sign may be a first sign of Duchenne muscular dystrophy (Escolar and Leshner, 2006)

If the rest of the examination has raised suspicion about muscle tone regulation and muscle power in the pelvic girdle or about the range of movements of the hip joints, these specific points of interest may be assessed in this position (or on an examination table).

Knee–heel test (Co)

Procedure (Figure 7.1)
The child is lying in supine. He is asked to put the heel of one foot on the knee of the other leg and to keep it there. After a few seconds, he is asked to move his heel down his leg towards the foot without losing contact with the leg. Instruction is facilitated when the examiner manually guides the first try out movement (Figures 7.1a and b). The child is told to place the heel as accurately as possible and to be careful when sliding it down. The child is not allowed to lift the head, i.e. the test should be performed in the absence of visual control. The test is repeated three times for each leg. It is advisable to count the number of performances achieved out loud and to provide continuous verbal guidance during the test. This prevents a 'slap dash' performance; which children often have a

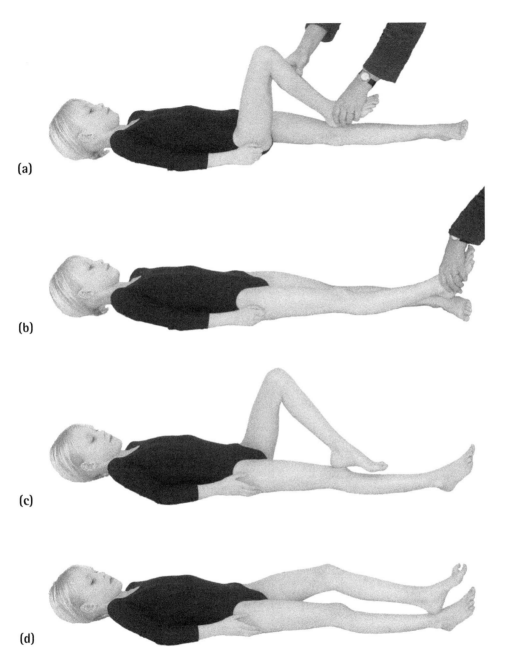

(a)

(b)

(c)

(d)

Figure 7.1 Knee–heel test in supine position. Instruction about how to perform the task includes demonstration: the examiner places the child's foot on the contralateral knee (a) and moves the foot slowly down along the lower leg to the foot (b). Next the child performs the task herself, three times with each leg (c) and (d). In between the tested leg should return to its resting position on the floor, i.e. the task does not consist of moving the heel up and down the lower leg.

preference for, but which precludes proper evaluation. When the child turns the test into an up and down sliding of the foot on the lower leg, the child is reminded that at the start the foot should be on the floor and next should 'fly' from that starting position through the air and land precisely on the knee.

Age

When clear instructions have been given the test is suitable for children aged 5 years and over. However, 5-year-olds do need substantial instruction and have some difficulties in placing and sliding. Children aged 6 and over are able to place the foot accurately on the knee and to produce a smooth and steady sliding movement of the foot.

Recording

Evaluation focuses on adequacy of foot placement and smoothness and accuracy of sliding. Each foot is assessed separately.

(1) Accurate placing is scored as follows:

   0 = typical, age-appropriate performance;

   1 = mildly abnormal;

   2 = definitely abnormal, serious difficulties in performance.

(2) Sliding heel is scored as follows:

   0 = typical, age-appropriate performance;

   1 = mildly abnormal;

   2 = definitely abnormal, serious difficulties in performance.

Asymmetries in performance are recorded. Mild abnormalities indicate the presence of one or two errors of placement or the presence of one or two slips of the leg during sliding. A definitely abnormal performance denotes the presence of a consistent failure to place the foot accurately, the presence of many slips, or the inability to keep the heel in contact with the lower leg.

Significance

This is a test of coordination of the legs in which cerebellar and proprioceptive functions play a part. Obviously weakness, hypotonia or hypertonia and hip deformities, or skeletal anomalies may also hamper an appropriate performance.

An intention tremor may be observed in severe cases of ataxia, but this condition falls outside the scope of this book.

Chapter 8
Assessment of the child sitting: part II

The child is asked to climb on the table again.

Assessment of processing of sensory information
As stressed in Chapter 3 (p. 13), specific use of classical neurological tests such as two-point discrimination, tactile sensation with cotton wool, or pain and temperature perception have not proved very useful in the neurological evaluation of children with suspected minor neurological dysfunction (MND), as the results are often unreliable. Nevertheless, during routine examination it is possible to make some general observations about the child's sensory functions. The examiner may note whether the child is excessively sensitive to touch.

Graphaesthesia (S)

PROCEDURE (FIGURE 8.1)
The examiner draws with her finger a cross or a circle in the palm of the child's hand and explains to the child that she will continue to draw crosses and circles and that the child has to feel what she draws. She asks the child to close his eyes. She draws a figure and asks the child after each drawing to report the nature of the figure felt. Each hand is tested with a random series of five drawings. The best cooperation is achieved when the test is performed in a 'train of trials', i.e. without pauses between the trials, so that the child's attention will not drift away. When the examiner hesitates and if poor performance is because of inattention or poor processing of sensory information some extra trials are performed.

AGE
The test is suitable for children of 5 years and over provided that the test is performed in an accurate and playful manner.

Figure 8.1 Graphaesthesia: the examiner draws a cross or a circle in the palm of the child's hand. The child has his eyes closed while the series of random crosses and circles are drawn.

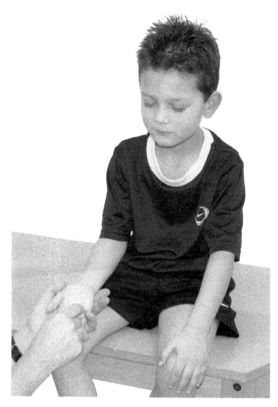

RECORDING
Performance is scored as follows:

> 0 = appropriate;
>
> 1 = inappropriate: R, L, R & L.

SIGNIFICANCE
Poor performance on the test of graphaesthesia may be of peripheral or central origin. With respect to the latter: the parietal cortex in particular plays a role in graphaesthesia.

Kinaesthesia (S)

PROCEDURE (FIGURE 8.2)
Evaluation for kinaesthesia is tested in both hands and feet. The assessment starts with the hands. The examiner takes the child's index finger between her thumb and index finger. Care is taken that the examiner's finger only touch the lateral parts of the child's finger in order to avoid additional pressure signals. The examiner moves the child's finger to and fro at the metacarpophalangeal joint while the rest of the child's hand and arm are kept still. The examiner explains that this is called 'movement'. Next she holds the finger still and explains that this is called 'still'. Explanation continues by telling the

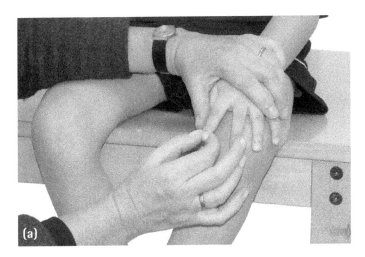

(a)

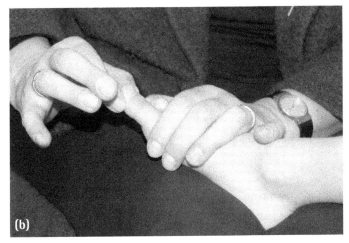

(b)

Figure 8.2 Starting position for kinaesthesia. (a) Hand: the examiner takes the child's index finger between her thumb and index finger in order to move it to and fro at the metacarpophalangeal joint. The rest of the upper extremity should be kept still, which can be achieved by placement of the child's hand on the child's knee. (b) Foot: the examiner takes the big toe between thumb and index finger and moves the toe to and fro at the metatarsalphalangeal joint. A good strategy to keep the rest of the foot and leg as still as possible is to put the child's foot on the examiner's lap.

child that a series of 'movements' and 'stills' will follow and that the child has to feel with closed eyes what is happening. Each hand is tested with a random series of five trials.

Testing of the feet follows. The examiner sits on a chair in front of the child with the child's foot on her lap. She takes the big toe between her thumb and index finger and takes care to touch the toe only laterally and to keep the rest of the foot and leg still when she moves the child's toe. The procedures that follow are similar to those used during testing of the hands. Each foot is tested with a random series of five trials.

Similar to the evaluation for graphaesthesia, the best cooperation is achieved when the test is performed in a 'train of trials', so that the child's attention does not drift away. When the examiner hesitates and if poor performance is as a result of inattention or poor processing of sensory information some extra trials are performed.

AGE
The test is suitable for children of 5 years and over provided that the test is performed in an accurate and playful manner.

RECORDING
Performance is scored as follows:

    0 = appropriate;
    1 = inappropriate: R, L, R & L.

SIGNIFICANCE
Poor performance may be of peripheral or central origin. Functional imaging studies revealed that in particular the frontal motor areas and the parietal primary and secondary sensory cortical areas are involved in the perception of passive movements (Radovanovic et al, 2002; Kavounoudias et al, 2008).

Sense of position (S)

PROCEDURE
The sense of position is evaluated in both hands and feet. The assessment starts with the hands. Procedures are largely comparable with those used during the evaluation of kinaesthesia (Figure 8.2). The examiner takes the child's index finger between her thumb and index finger. Care is taken that the examiner's finger only touches the lateral parts of the child's finger in order to avoid additional pressure signals. The examiner moves the child's finger to and fro at the metacarpophalangeal joint while the rest of the child's hand and arm are kept still. Then she holds the finger in an extreme position and explains to the child that this is called pointing 'to you' (or what ever the finger points to). In a similar way another extreme position is labelled. Explanation continues by telling the child that a series of positions will follow and that the child has to feel with closed eyes which direction the finger is pointing. Each hand is tested with a random series of five trials.

Testing of the feet follows. The examiner sits on a chair in front of the child with the child's foot on her lap. She takes the big toe between her thumb and index finger and takes care to touch the toe only laterally and to keep the rest of the foot and leg still when she moves the child's toe. The steps that follow are similar to those used during testing of the hands. Each foot is tested with a random series of five trials.

Similar to evaluations of the other sensory modalities the best cooperation is achieved when the test is performed in a 'train of trials', so that the child's attention does not drift away. When the examiner hesitates and if poor performance is as a result of inattention or poor processing of sensory information some extra trials are performed.

AGE
The test is suitable for children of 5 years and over provided that the test is performed in an accurate and playful manner.

RECORDING
Performance is scored as follows:

0 = appropriate;
1 = inappropriate: R, L, R & L.

SIGNIFICANCE
Poor performance may be of peripheral or central, in particular parietal, origin.

Facial motility (CN)

PROCEDURE (FIGURE 8.3)
The examiner must observe the facial musculature at rest and then during voluntary and emotional movements. For this purpose, the child is asked to show his teeth, frown, blow out his cheeks, whistle and then close his eyes.

AGE
The tests are suitable for children of 4 years and over provided that questions are asked in a playful manner. Children below 9 years often have problems in producing a whistling sound; they can, however produce a 'whistling face'.

RECORDING
Performance is scored as follows:

    0 = typical;
    1 = abnormal: R, L, R & L.

SIGNIFICANCE
Unilateral peripheral facial palsies show an asymmetry in both upper and lower parts of the face, whereas a supranuclear lesion shows ipsilateral asymmetry, especially in the lower parts of the face. In these cases, the facial musculature during emotional movements may be relatively less affected. However, when a nuclear or peripheral lesion is involved the face is affected at all times.

It is often difficult to assess the symmetry or asymmetry of the neuromuscular functioning of the facial musculature, as many children may have a somewhat asymmetrically shaped skull and face. It may occasionally be necessary to measure the distance between the lateral corner of the eye and the corner of the mouth on each side of the face, and the distance between the ear and the corner of the mouth. It is always worth inspecting the child's head from above to detect any sign of plagiocephaly that might influence the symmetry of the face. From the age of 4, some children may develop habitual, often asymmetrical, features without any clear neurological significance.

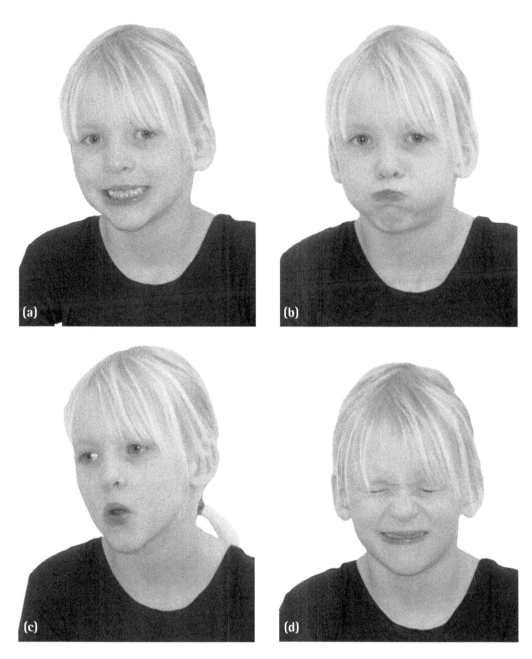

Figure 8.3 Facial movement is observed throughout the assessment and during some 'on demand' voluntary activities, such as (a) 'show your teeth', (b) 'blow out your cheeks', (c) 'whistle', and (d) 'close your eyes tightly'. Special attention is paid to symmetry of movement.

Eyes

Visual acuity (S)

RECORDING OF USE OF VISUAL CORRECTION, E.G. SPECTACLES
This is recorded as follows:

    0 = no need for correction;
    1 = need for positive lenses (note diopters);
    2 = need for negative glasses (note diopters).

SIGNIFICANCE
Refractive errors, like strabismus, are often found in children who had a complicated perinatal history, such as a preterm birth (O'Connor and Fielder, 2007; Evensen et al, 2009). Clear neurological impairment, such as cerebral palsy, is also associated with the presence of myopia, hyperopia, and astigmatism (Mackie et al, 1998). The association between neurological impairment and refractive errors supports the notion that central visual feedback mechanisms play a role in the growth of the eye (Flitcroft et al, 2005).

Position of the eyes (CN)

PROCEDURE
The examiner must look for concomitant or non-concomitant strabismus. Slight squints may be detected by looking for symmetry of the corneal reflections. The 'cover test' may be used to detect latent strabismus or heterophoria; each eye is covered in turn while the child looks at a distant object (which does not require convergence). A slight movement may be observed in the uncovered eye either immediately after the other eye is covered, or more often in the covered eye when the cover is removed. The slight movements are often best seen by looking at the corneal reflections. This test is based on the fact that in heterophoria, external eye muscle activity is needed to prevent diplopia, even when the eyes are 'resting'. When one eye is covered, this necessity disappears and the eye muscles can relax. As soon as the cover is removed, contraction of one or more of the eye muscles becomes necessary again, manifesting itself as a slight movement of the eye. The eye that shows movements is the eye with heterophoria. Latent strabismus is a frequently occurring condition, which becomes more evident when the child is tired. Therefore, it is advisable to take into account the time of the day at which the assessment takes place, and the other activities the child has been involved in that day.

When the eye drifts towards the temporal side the condition is called exophoria; to the nasal side, esophoria; upwards, hyperphoria; and downwards, hypophoria. If the eye muscles are not able to bring the visual axes to bear upon the same point, squint or strabismus is present (exotropia, esotropia, hypertropia or hypotropia respectively). In this event, the only way to avoid diplopia is to suppress one image, which leads to a reduction of visual acuity in the squinting eye.

AGE
The position of the eyes can be assessed from infancy onwards.

RECORDING
The presence or absence of heterophoria, concomitant strabismus or non-concomitant strabismus must be recorded. Where present, the eye involved and the type of heterophoria or squint must be described. In the case of non-concomitant strabismus, the eye muscles involved must be described by observing the movements the child is able to make when following an object in his visual field. These should be scored as follows:

0 = typical;
1 = heterophoria: R, L, R & L;
2 = convergent strabismus: R, L, R & L;
3 = otherwise abnormal.

SIGNIFICANCE
The detection of heterophoria is most important since its presence may hamper the child's ability in close work such as reading, drawing, and writing; the muscular strain required leading to fatigue. An accurate estimate of visual acuity is an essential part of assessing how much the eye has deteriorated as a result of a manifest strabismus; in such cases, there is usually an impairment of visual acuity in one eye, especially in children aged 5 and over. However, amblyopia ex anopsia (stimulus-deprivation amblyopia) does not necessarily occur in children aged 3 or 4, since these children often use both eyes alternately (i.e. alternate monocular vision).

In true concomitant strabismus, the angle between the two axes should remain constant over the entire range of eye movements, although this need not be exactly the case. Concomitant strabismus may be due to peripheral i.e. ophthalmological or central neural dysfunction but the cause is often unknown, especially in the case of congenital strabismus. A hereditary factor is often present, although it may also be found in children with a history of perinatal adversity or short gestation.

In non-concomitant strabismus the angle between the eye axes changes according to the direction of the gaze. In mild cases the strabismus may disappear when the eye is looking in one direction but it will then be maximal in the gaze direction opposite to that position. For example in the case of a (mild) abducens paresis (VIth cranial nerve) of the left eye, the strabismus will be minimal or even absent on looking to the left side, i.e. to the side of the paretic muscle. Non-concomitant strabismus may result from ocular paresis caused by a number of conditions (e.g. congenital or traumatic factors, disease of the orbita, toxins, infectious diseases, diseases of the central nervous system, or eye muscle diseases). Of particular interest is a generally benign and often transient paresis of the VIth cranial nerve some weeks after an otitis media or upper respiratory infection. A paresis of the ocular muscles of long standing may eventually result in a concomitant strabismus.

Fixation (CN)

PROCEDURE (FIGURE 8.4)
The child is asked to focus on an object (such as the point of a pencil, the handle of the reflex hammer, or a little figure) that is held in front of his eyes for 15 seconds at a distance of about 40 cm. Three aspects are considered: deviations of one or both eyes; choreiform movements (i.e. jerky movements of both eyes that occur irregularly and arrhythmically in all directions); and manifest strabismus. Also the presence of choreiform movements in the face during this test is noted.

AGE
Fixation can be assessed from infancy onwards.

RECORDING
Deviations, choreiform movements, and squint are recorded as absent or present, and the involved eye and direction of the deviation or squint are specified. The deviations in position are recorded in the item 'position of the eyes'.

(1)   Choreiform movements of the eyes (Ch) are scored as follows:

    0 = absent;

    1 = presence of an occasional choreiform movement (+);

    2 = frequently occurring choreiform movements (++).

(2)   Choreiform movements of the face (Ch) are scored as follows:

    0 = absent;

    1 = presence of an occasional choreiform movement (+);

    2 = frequently occurring choreiform movements (++).

SIGNIFICANCE
Deviation of one eye during fixation may be the result of latent strabismus (heterophoria) or to an ocular paresis (see position of the eyes test above). The significance of choreiform movements is discussed in Chapter 5 (p. 59).

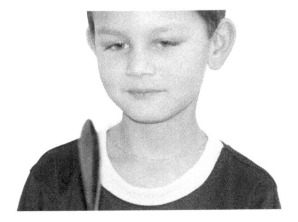

Figure 8.4 Visual fixation: the child is asked to fixate an object that is held in front of his eyes for 15 seconds at a distance of about 40 cm.

Pupillary reactions (CN)

PROCEDURE (FIGURE 8.5)
The size of the pupil is noted and then a bright light is flashed into one eye only and the reactions of both pupils observed. The easiest way to prevent a direct light stimulus in the contralateral eye is to put the examiner's hand as a barrier between the eyes. The procedure is repeated with the other eye. The child should be in such a position that light from outside or from a ceiling light falls on both eyes equally.

AGE
Pupillary reactions can be assessed at any age.

RECORDING
Performance should be scored as follows:

  0 = typical and symmetrical direct and indirect reactions;
  1 = abnormal: R, L, R & L.

Pupillary reactions may be absent, slow, or fast. If a light is flashed into one eye (direct reaction), the contralateral pupil (indirect reaction) should contract simultaneously with the stimulated pupil.

SIGNIFICANCE
Reaction to light should be prompt and marked. No contraction of the pupils may be the result of peripheral or central causes. A negative indirect reaction results from unilateral blindness, caused by a lesion of the optic nerve. A weak and slow contraction may be as a result of drugs, infections, post-infectious conditions or a generalized depression of nervous functions. For a more elaborated discussion on pupillary reactions the reader is referred to textbooks on paediatric neurology and neurophysiology.

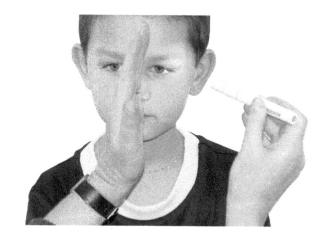

Figure 8.5 Pupillary reactions: the size of the pupil is noted and then a bright light is flashed into one eye only and the narrowing reactions of both pupils observed. The examiner's hand prevents a direct light stimulus of the contralateral eye.

Visual pursuit movements, including convergence (CN)

PROCEDURE (FIGURE 8.6)
The examiner moves a little figure, a pencil, or the reflex hammer in front of the child at a moderate tempo in both the horizontal and the vertical plane. Then convergence is tested by moving the object from a distance of about 50 cm towards the nose of the child.

The child is asked to follow the object with his eyes, keeping his head still. In general children find it hard to keep their head still; instead they move their head in the direction of the moving object. When this occurs the examiner stabilizes the child's head with a light touch of her hand.

Two aspects are assessed: the quality and the range of the ocular movements. Movements may be smooth, jerky, ataxic, or choreiform. The last category is used for vertical jerky movements when the eyes move sideways, and horizontal jerky movements when the eyes move upwards and downwards, occurring simultaneously in both eyes.

AGE
Visual pursuit can be assessed from infancy onwards.

RECORDING
(1) Pursuit movements of the eyes are scored as follows:

   0 = typical in all directions;

   1 = abnormal: movements in all directions, but jerky quality (jerks in the direction of the pursuit movement);

   2 = abnormal: imbalance of the eyes;

   3 = abnormal: movements limited in specific directions (describe this).

(2) Choreiform movements of the eyes during pursuit (Ch) are scored as follows:

   0 = absent;

   1 = presence of an occasional choreiform movement (+);

   2 = frequently occurring choreiform movements (++).

(3) Choreiform movements of the face during pursuit (Ch) are scored as follows:

   0 = absent;

   1 = presence of an occasional choreiform movement (+);

   2 = frequently occurring choreiform movements (++).

(4) Nystagmus (CN) is scored as follows:

   0 = bilaterally absent;

   1 = unilaterally present: R, L;

   2 = bilaterally present.

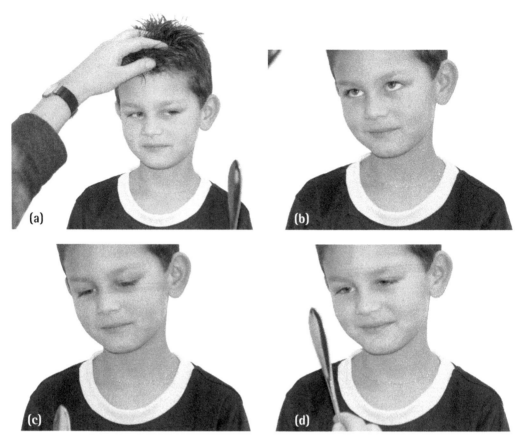

Figure 8.6 Visual pursuit: the examiner moves an object in front of the child in a moderate tempo to the (a) left, to the right (not shown in figure), (b) upwards, (c) downwards, and (d) towards the nose of the child to test convergence.

Any abnormalility in the ability to follow the object is described and any restriction of the full range of movements is recorded. Choreiform and jerky eye movements are noted. During this test the examiner should also ascertain the presence of concomitant or non-concomitant strabismus, and in the latter case, which muscles are involved (Table 8.1). In children with latent strabismus (but apparently also independent of that condition) a type of 'imbalance' of the eyes may be present. During following a moving object the eye axes of both eyes remain parallel over the range of movements, but this parallelism is lost at the end and beginning of the movement. This is seen particularly during the return movements after looking sideways. One eye seems to change its movement pattern faster than the other eye, which may even give the impression of remaining static, while the first eye moves. Usually the contralateral eye (i.e. the eye in the nasal position) remains static or moves less.

Attention is paid to the presence of nystagmus. Nystagmus consists of involuntary oscillatory eye movements, usually with a slow and a rapid component. The latter is

Table 8.1 Action of individual eye muscles

Eye muscle	Action	Cranial nerve
Lateral rectus	To the temporal side	Abducens nerve (VI)
Medial rectus	To the nasal side	Oculomotor nerve (III)
Superior rectus	Upwards and slightly inwards	Oculomotor nerve (III)
Inferior rectus	Downwards and slightly inwards	Oculomotor nerve (III)
Inferior oblique	Upwards and slightly outwards	Oculomotor nerve (III)
Superior oblique	Downwards and slightly outwards	Trochlear nerve (IV)

used to give the direction of the nystagmus. Nystagmus may be observed during fixation, this is the so-called spontaneous nystagmus. A nystagmus that occurs first at the extreme positions of the eyes is called a directional nystagmus. When a nystagmus is observed, the character (spontaneous or directional) is recorded and the direction of the rapid component described if present. The intensity of the nystagmus should also be described and a note made of any asymmetries.

SIGNIFICANCE
Deviations in the visual pursuit of an object may be the result of paresis of the ocular muscles. Diplopia is rarely found in children because of rapid cortical suppression of one image. The significance of choreiform movements is discussed in Chapter 5 (p. 59).

'Imbalance' can be a sign of latent strabismus, but seems to exist without heterophoria. Its presence is often associated with other signs of MND. However, its significance for reading difficulties is not well understood.

A horizontal, pendular nystagmus, which is present from shortly after birth, is called 'congenital nystagmus'. Its aetiology is obscure; the intensity may be affected by the position of the head. Nearly always, vision is impaired. Spontaneous non-congenital nystagmus may be the result of disturbances of the vestibular system, which may be of infectious, toxic, traumatic, or other origin. In most cases, directional nystagmus is of vestibular origin but it may be as a result of functional weakness of the eye muscles.

Visual field (S)

PROCEDURE (FIGURE 8.7)
The examiner manoeuvres herself so that the face of the child and her own face are at the same level. She asks the child to fixate on her nose (or a small object held about 40 cm in front of the child). Then she moves a small object or for example a reflex hammer from behind the child's head so that it gradually enters his visual field on one side. The child is instructed to grasp the object as soon as he catches sight of it. The test is carried out from each side and from above the child's head. By being positioned immediately in front of the child, the examiner is able to observe whether the child fixates well. Eager to

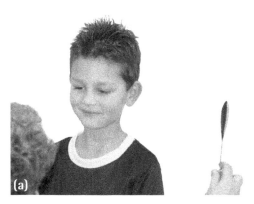

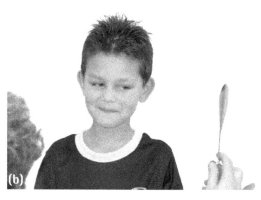

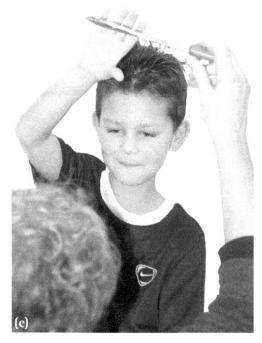

Figure 8.7 Evaluation of visual fields. The face of the child and the examiner are at the same level. (a) The child fixates on the examiner's nose, while the examiner moves an object from behind the child's head so that it gradually enters his visual field. (b) Evaluation of the lateral visual field: the child grasps the object as soon as he sees the object. This is accompanied by a visual orientation response. (c) Evaluation of the upper visual fields.

perform well children are inclined to 'peep', i.e. they tend to direct visual attention early during the manoeuvre towards the tested direction. When 'peeping' is observed, the child is gently reminded to fixate on the central target. Children usually are surprised that the examiner notices the 'peeping' and tend to fixate well after the 'magic' feedback of the examiner.

The procedure allows a crude impression of the child's visual fields. The test can be repeated with objects of different sizes and colours.

AGE
The test is suitable for children of 5 years and over.

RECORDING
Performance is scored as follows:

> 0 = typical;
> 1 = abnormal, R, L eye, R & L eyes.

The normal angle of vision to the side is between 60° and 80° and above is about 45°. It is often unnecessary to wait for actual grasping. Usually an orienting response occurs as soon as the object enters the visual field, and that causes a movement of the eye towards the stimulus. Presence of this orienting is sufficient for a positive score on this test.

SIGNIFICANCE
The most common visual field defects in children are homonymous hemianopia, which generally accompanies spastic hemiplegia, and bitemporal hemianopia resulting from tumours near the optic chiasm, which may arise quite insidiously. Lesser defects, such as quadrantic defects of the visual fields, are rare (deriving from craniopharyngioma or a temporal lobe tumour involving optic radiation). Although such cases evidently surpass the bounds of minor dysfunction, a visual field defect may be the first clinical sign. The above test is sufficient for routine purposes, but if there is any doubt, perimetry should be carried out; however, this may be rather difficult and unreliable in children below the age of 6 or 7.

The examiner must bear in mind that diminished visual acuity may be responsible for diminished visual fields. As with other tests of visuo-ocular abilities, any abnormal findings warrant referral to an ophthalmologist.

EARS

Hearing

PROCEDURE
The examiner sits or stands about 5.5 m (6 yards) away from the child and in a low voice pronounces test words of different sound spectra ('66', '100', '99') including single consonantal sounds ('sss', 'rrr', 'mmm') and vowel sounds ('uuuu', 'aaaa'). Each ear is tested in turn, the child keeping the other ear covered with his hand and repeating the sounds as heard.

AGE
The test is suitable for children aged 4 and over.

RECORDING
Scoring of deficits is as follows:

> 0 = no;
> 1 = yes: R, L, R & L.

SIGNIFICANCE
A dubious response indicates the need for further audiological examination.

MOUTH

Tongue

PROCEDURE
The child is asked to stick out his tongue and keep it as still as possible. After about 10 seconds, voluntary movements of discomfort may occur. Any occurrence of involuntary movements should be carefully noted. Next the child is asked to move his tongue from side to side, touching the corners of his mouth. Subsequently he is asked to move his tongue along his teeth in the upper and lower jaws in a near circular movement. Finally, he is asked to protrude it as far as possible.

AGE
The test is suitable for children of 5 years and over.

RECORDING
(1) Tongue motility (CN) is scored as follows:
    0 = typical;
    1 = abnormal.
(2) Choreiform movements of the tongue (Ch) are scored as follows:
    0 = absent;
    1 = presence of an occasional choreiform movement (+);
    2 = frequently occurring choreiform movements (++).

SIGNIFICANCE
Children of 5 years and over should be able to move their tongue smoothly from side to side and to keep the tongue still in protrusion. Awkwardness of tongue movements, and also drooling, which is often a sign of disturbances of swallowing, may be related to speech difficulties. A short frenulum of the tongue, in the majority of cases, is of little clinical significance.

A discussion of the significance of choreiform and athetoid movements can be found in Chapter 5 (p. 59). Choreiform movements must be differentiated from fasciculations. Choreiform movements occur in more extended areas of the tongue and lead to gross movements. Fasciculations are asynchronous, irregular, rapid twitches of very small parts of the tongue. The tongue is the only muscle in which fasciculations can be observed, myograms being necessary for other muscles. Fasciculations are generally a sign of a serious, progressive disease (e.g. bulbar disorders).

Pharyngeal arches

PROCEDURE (FIGURE 8.8)
The child is asked to open his mouth as wide as possible so that the examiner can inspect the pharyngeal arches at rest. Then the child is asked to say 'aaaa' so that the examiner may inspect them during movement. The use of a penlight facilitates inspection.

AGE
The test is suitable for children aged 4 and over.

RECORDING
This is scored as follows:

   0 = symmetrical, typical;
   1 = asymmetrical.

SIGNIFICANCE
Asymmetries of the pharyngeal arches, particularly during phonation, may be related to difficulties in speech and speech development. However, for several weeks or even months after tonsillectomy, some children may show temporary asymmetry of movement of the arches, without evident impairment of speech or swallowing.

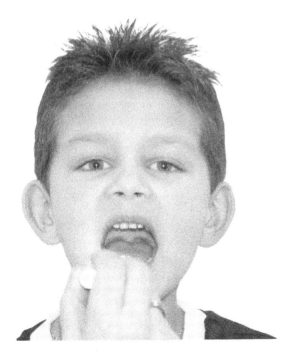

Figure 8.8 Assessment of motility of the pharyngeal arches during production of 'aaa' sound.

Chapter 9
General data

When the assessment of the head has been concluded, the neurological examination is virtually completed. However, there are certain aspects of a general paediatric and developmental examination that may yield important information to the neurologist. For instance, the relationship between the child's weight and his height is relevant to an assessment of the quality of movement, since an overweight child may show a different quality of movement to that of a child of slender build. For example, an obese child will often show a slower speed of movement, whereas a slender child may be more agile. In the case of clumsiness this difference may result in different phenotypical behaviour, for instance show coarse and awkward movement patterns versus very fast, abrupt and 'hurry-scurry' motor behaviour. It is useful, therefore, to weigh and measure the child, and also to measure the circumference of the skull (for micro- or macrocephaly) and to describe any abnormalities in the shape of the skull (for plagiocephaly, synostosis of a single suture, etc.).

In addition to anthropometric data, quantity and quality of spontaneous motor behaviour, somatognosis, and hand preference are assessed.

Quantity of spontaneous motor activity

Procedure
The quantity of spontaneous motor activity during the entire assessment is recorded; both small and gross movements are taken into account.

Age
The quantity of movement can be evaluated at any age.

Recording
Performance is scored as follows:

0 = typical;
1 = abnormal, decreased (↓) or increased (↑).

Significance
The quantity of spontaneous motor activity varies greatly from individual to individual. Yet, the consistent presence of a low or high level of spontaneous activity during the assessment is noteworthy. Very little spontaneous activity (hypokinesia) in general is an indication of illness, usually an acute illness. Its presence means that the neurological assessment should be postponed to another occasion. A high level of spontaneous activity (hyperkinesia) during the assessment may be an indication of attention-deficit–hyperactivity disorder (ADHD).

Quality of spontaneous motor activity

Procedure
The quality of spontaneous motor activity during the entire assessment is recorded; both fine and gross motor behaviour is taken into account.

Age
The quality of movement can be evaluated at any age.

Recording
Performance is scored as follows:

0 = typical;
1 = abnormal (describe).

Significance
The quality of motor behaviour is a sensitive marker of neural function (Prechtl, 2001). Minor neurological dysfunction (MND) is often associated with an abnormal quality of movement. Examples of movements with an atypical quality are jerky, abrupt, sluggish, stiff, awkward, poorly organized, or stereotyped movements.

Somatognosis – knowledge of body schema

Procedure
The examiner asks the child whether he knows various body parts by asking questions such as 'Where is your nose?', 'Where is your elbow?'. Next she asks the child if he knows what is left and right. If the child has some knowledge of left and right, the child is asked to indicate where for instance the left thumb or the right foot is. If the child has an adequate knowledge of right and left, the child is asked to perform various

movements during which the child has to cross the midline and also some movements without crossing the midline. An example of a crossing movement is 'Can you point with your right index finger to your left cheek?'; an example of a non-crossing movement is 'Can you put your left hand on your left knee?'.

Age
Children of 4 years and over have an adequate knowledge of the various parts of the body. From age 5 onwards children also should know their left and right. The task with crossing and non-crossing movements is more complex; from 7 onwards children can usually cope with this task.

Recording
(1) Basic knowledge of body parts is scored as follows:

  0 = age-appropriate performance;
  1 = inappropriate performance.
(2) Knowledge of left and right is scored as follows:

  0 = age-appropriate performance;
  1 = inappropriate performance.
(3) Crossing/non-crossing the midline is scored as follows:

  0 = age-appropriate performance;
  1 = inappropriate performance.

Significance
Knowledge of the body has a widespread cortical representation, in which the parietal cortex plays a prominent role (Njiokiktjien, 2007).

Hand preference

Procedure
The child is asked which hand he uses in general for writing, drawing, cutting with scissors and using a spoon. When the child does not provide a clear answer, the child is asked to draw or write, to cut a piece of paper and to tap with a (reflex) hammer on the table. The necessary implements are handed to the child in a neutral position, with no bias to right or left.

Age
From the age of 4 onwards most children show a clear preference for either the right or left hand.

Recording
This is scored as follows:

  0 = right;
  1 = left;
  2 = ambidextrous, i.e. mixed handedness.

Significance
About 85% of adults have a preference for the right hand, 10% have a preference for the left, and 4% are ambidextrous (Perelle and Ehrman, 1994). It is important to appreciate that hand preference is not the same as 'dominance'. The latter term is generally used to imply something about neurological organization, suggesting that one hemisphere is superior to the other in controlling particular motor functions.

During prenatal life fetuses in general show a preference for the right side of the body, i.e. in the second and third trimester of gestation the right arm is moved more frequently than the left (McCartney and Hepper, 1999). Near-term age fetuses and preterm infants also develop a slight preference for turning the head to the right side (Vles and Van Oostenbrugge, 1988; Ververs et al, 1994). But during the first postnatal year infant motor behaviour is characterized in particular by variation, including variable hand use (Touwen, 1993; Hadders-Algra, 2000a). The hand preference of infants is inconsistent and may change on a daily or weekly base (Corbetta and Thelen, 1996). During the preschool years, hand preference gradually becomes more consistent and reaches a relatively stable pattern between 3 and 4 years of age (Gesell and Ames, 1947; Hempel, 1993a and 1993b).

For many decades it was thought that handedness was mainly determined by genetic factors (Annett, 1979). Recent studies, however, indicate that handedness is brought about by complex interactions between genetic information and environmental influences. The latter include prenatal and perinatal risk factors, asymmetrical perception during early postnatal life induced by asymmetrical head position or parental care, and social and cultural modulation (Schaafsma et al, 2009). The role of early environmental factors is illustrated by the association between preterm birth and left handedness (Marlow et al, 1989; O'Callaghan et al,1993) and between prenatal stress and extremely preterm birth (gestational age at birth ≤25 weeks) and mixed handedness (Marlow et al, 2007; Rodriguez and Waldenström, 2008). Non-right handedness is not only associated with prenatal and perinatal adversities, but also with an increased prevalence of neurodevelopmental disorders: mixed handedness is associated with language problems, ADHD (Rodriguez and Waldenström, 2008), and schizophrenia (Cannon et al, 1995), and left handedness with developmental coordination disorder (DCD; Goez and Zelnik 2008). The associations between handedness and prenatal and perinatal risk factors and neurodevelopmental impairment underscore the relevance of inclusion of the assessment of handedness in a neurodevelopmental assessment.

Chapter 10

Interpretation of findings

Introduction: MND in the framework of the *International Classification of Functioning, Disability and Health: Children and Youth version*

When a child has been referred to a clinic because of motor impairments interfering with activities of daily life, a learning and/or a behavioural disorder, the assessment consists of the evaluation of the child's prenatal, perinatal and developmental history, the history of the current problems, the social and family history, and various specialist assessments, including a paediatric assessment. The battery of assessments may include a psychological assessment, a psychiatric assessment, a motor assessment (e.g. the Movement ABC, Henderson and Sugden, 2007), an assessment of handwriting, a speech and language assessment, or a behavioural assessment by means of questionnaires. A neurological assessment evaluating the presence of minor neurological dysfunction (MND) is recommended (see Chapter 2).

The series of assessments results in a biopsychosocial profile of the child that can be interpreted in terms of the *International Classification of Functioning, Disability and Health: Children and Youth version* (ICF–CY, World Health Organization, 2007; Figure 10.1). The ICF–CY has two parts to it: functioning and disability; and contextual factors. Functioning and disability are described from three perspectives: (1) body functions/impairments; (2) activity/activity limitations; and (3) participation/participation restrictions. In this model environmental factors such as assistive technology, attitudes, and services belong to the contextual part. The examination of MND is a tool addressing body function. The ICF–CY model underscores the notion that body function is only one of the factors determining activity and participation i.e. one of the factors that for instance determine whether behaviour or motor impairments result in activity limitation or restriction of participation.

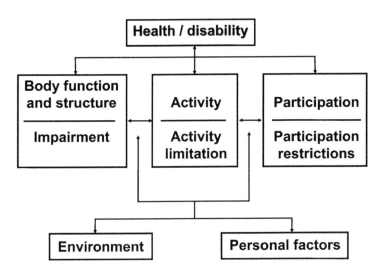

Figure 10.1 The International Classification of Functioning, Disability and Health: Children and Youth Version (WHO, 2007). The classification can be used to describe interactions between different constructs and domains by providing a multidisciplinary approach to function and disability. Figure used with permission from WHO.

Interpretation of neurological findings

The neurological examination must be followed by an interpretation of the neurological findings. The significance of the findings can only be evaluated after the comprehensive and descriptive examination is completed, i.e. when the examiner tries to see if the neurological data can be fitted into a meaningful pattern. The interpretation of findings should follow the following rules for decision-making.

(1) Do the findings fit into a 'classical' pattern of neurological findings, for instance into the configuration of signs of cerebral palsy? The latter implies for instance, in the case of bilateral spastic cerebral palsy, the combination of a stereotyped posture and movement of the legs, increased muscle tone and brisk tendon reflexes in the legs, and Babinski signs. Criteria for the diagnosis of the various forms of cerebral palsy have been described by Platt et al (2009).

  • If the answer is 'yes', a clinical neurological diagnosis is established. Findings in terms of MND may be used in addition to findings in the least affected parts of the body, for instance of the least affected side of the body in a child with a unilateral spastic cerebral palsy.

  • If the answer is 'no', a description of the child's neurological profile in terms of domains of dysfunctions follows (see 2). The neurological profile in terms of MND is not a classical neurological diagnosis,[1] but provides information about the strengths and weaknesses of the child's brain function.

---

1 Diagnostics in terms of minor neurological dysfunction frequently have been a source of misunderstanding and debate. This is reflected by labelling 'soft neurological signs' as a marker of 'soft thinking' (Ingram, 1973; Touwen and Sporrel, 1979) and the neurologist applying the concept of soft signs as a 'soft neurologist' (Stephenson, 2001). To avoid misperception and the connotation of imprecise definition and malleability Touwen and Prechtl (1970; Touwen, 1979) introduced the consistent use of the term minor neurological dysfunction instead of 'soft signs'.

(2) Description of the neurological profile: domains of dysfunction. The studies on soft signs and MND revealed that a perfect brain is an exception rather than a rule (Tupper, 1987). Many children (and adults) show single signs of dysfunction in one or more of the eight neurological domains. Isolated signs of dysfunction have, however, limited clinical significance (cf. Hadders-Algra et al, 1988c; Breslau et al, 2000; Fellick et al, 2001). Therefore threshold criteria for dysfunction in the various domains of dysfunction have been determined (Box 10.1 and Table 10.1). The child's neurological performance in the eight domains constitutes the child's neurological profile. The profile provides information on the severity and the type of MND.

The severity of dysfunction is expressed by its classification into a normal neurological condition, simple MND, and complex MND. At school age (from 4 years until the onset of puberty) classification is determined by the number of domains of dysfunction, after the onset of puberty the type of dysfunction is critical (Table 10.2). The latter also means that after the onset of puberty the distinction between severity and type of dysfunction fades. At school age a child is classified as having a simple MND when one or two domains are dysfunctional and as having a complex MND when more than two domains are dysfunctional. After the onset of puberty the isolated presence of dysfunctional posture and muscle tone regulation, mild dyskinesia, excessive associated movements, sensory dysfunction, and mild cranial nerve dysfunction results in the classification of simple MND and the presence of mild coordination problems or fine manipulative disability in complex MND. At any age, a normal neurological condition is denoted by the absence of dysfunctional domains or the isolated presence of dysfunction in the domain of reflexes. The latter means that abnormal reflex activity only has clinical significance when it is accompanied by neurological signs in other domains. The lack of clinical significance of the isolated presence of dysfunction in the domain of reflexes is related to the variable behaviour of reflexes over time, a characteristic which reflects a genuine property of the nervous system (Stam and Van Crevel, 1989).

Box 10.1 Domains of dysfunction based on the functional neurobehavioural subsystems of the nervous system (Hadders–Algra et al, 1988c; Peters et al, 2008)

- Dysfunctional posture and muscle tone regulation.
- Dysfunctional reflex activity.
- Mild dyskinesia, e.g. choreiform dyskinesia, athetotiform dyskinesia.
- Mild problems in coordination.
- Mild problems in fine manipulative ability.
- Excessive associated movements.
- Mild cranial nerve dysfunction.
- Mild sensory dysfunction.

Table 10.1 Criteria for dysfunction per domain (see Peters et al, 2008)

Domain	Based on	Criteria for the presence of a dysfunctional domain
(1) Posture and muscle tone	Posture during sitting, standing and walking Muscle tone	Two or more of the following: mild deviations of muscle tone in legs mild deviations of muscle tone in arms consistent mild deviations in posture
(2) Reflexes	Intensity tendon reflexes arms: high, low or asymmetrical Threshold tendon reflexes arms: high, low or asymmetrical Intensity tendon reflexes legs: high, low or asymmetrical Threshold tendon reflexes legs: high, low or asymmetrical Footsole response: uni- or bilateral Babinski sign Plantar grasp: uni- or bilaterally present Abdominal skin reflex: asymmetry	Presence of at least two signs
(3) Involuntary movements	Spontaneous motor behaviour Test for involuntary movements Movements of face, eyes, tongue	Presence of at least one of following: marked, consistent choreiform movements of distal muscles marked, consistent choreiform movements of proximal muscles marked choreiform movements of face, eyes and/or tongue marked, consistent tremor consistent athetotiform movements in distal muscles
(4) Coordination and balance	Finger–nose test Fingertip–touching test Diadochokinesis Kicking Knee–heel test Reaction to push, sitting Reaction to push, standing Romberg test	Three or more tests inappropriate for age

Table 10.1 Continued

Domain	Based on	Criteria for the presence of a dysfunctional domain
	Walking along a straight line Standing on one leg Hopping on one leg	
(5) Fine manipulation	Finger opposition test: smoothness Finger opposition test: transition Follow-a-finger test Circle test	Two or more test-items inappropriate for age
(6) Associated movements	Associated movements during: diadochokinesis finger opposition test walking on toes walking on heels mouth-opening and finger-spreading phenomenon	Presence of an excessive amount of associated movements for age in at least three tests
(7) Sensory function	Graphaesthesia Kinaesthesia Sense of position Hearing Visual fields	Two or more sensory functions dysfunctional
(8) Cranial nerve function	Motor behaviour of face, eyes, pharynx, and tongue	Mild cranial nerve palsy

Simple and complex MND
For many years the high prevalence of signs of MND and the limited clinical significance of single signs blurred the clinical value of identifying MND (Kennard, 1960; Barlow 1974; Nichols and Chen, 1981; Tupper, 1987). However, the distinction of two basic forms of MND, i.e. simple and complex MND, helped to clarify the picture.

Simple MND
Simple MND has a high prevalence. Figures from the Groningen Perinatal Project of children born in the 1970s indicated that about 15% of school-age children showed simple MND (Hadders-Algra, 2002), but a recent study of children born in the late 1990s suggested that the prevalence of simple MND in children attending mainstream primary education in the Netherlands is about 20% (Peters et al, 2010). The high prevalence of simple MND and its weak association with prenatal, perinatal, and neonatal adversities suggest that the simple form of MND belongs to the spectrum of typical neurological conditions. In other words, simple MND may be regarded as a minor neurological

Table 10.2 Criteria for simple and complex minor neurological dysfunction (MND; see Hadders–Algra, 2002)

Age	Critical in classification	Simple MND	Complex MND
4 years until the onset of puberty[a]	Number of dysfunctional domains	Presence of 1[b] or 2 dysfunctional domains	Presence of >2 dysfunctional domains
After the onset of puberty	Type of dysfunctional domain	Isolated presence of: dysfunctional posture and tone regulation choreiform dyskinesia excessive associated movements mild sensory dysfunction mild cranial nerve dysfunction	Presence of: mild coordination problems fine manipulative disability (with or without other domains of dysfunction)

a. Onset of puberty: presence of clear physical expression of puberty (Soorani-Lunsing et al, 1993).
b. One exception to the rule: the isolated presence of a dysfunctional domain in 'reflexes' does not qualify for the classification 'simple minor dysfunctional disorders' but denotes the presence of a normal neurological condition.

difference. Most likely it represents typical but non-optimal brain function. The aetiology of simple MND is largely unknown. Presumably, genetic information is a major determinant of simple MND. However, prenatal, perinatal, and neonatal risk factors may play an additional role. Interestingly, the factors that have been associated with an increased risk for simple MND or a non-optimal neurological condition, such as preterm birth without serious neonatal complications, severe intrauterine growth retardation without signs of fetal distress, an Apgar score at 3 minutes below seven, and maternal anxiety during pregnancy (Ley et al, 1996; Hadders-Algra, 2002; Fallang et al, 2005; Arnaud et al, 2007; Kikkert et al, 2010), are associated with stress during early life. Data from animal studies indicate that stress during early ontogeny gives rise to changes in serotonergic and noradrenergic activity in the cerebral cortex and alterations in dopaminergic activity in the striatum and prefrontal cortex (Weinstock, 2001). However, in humans it is not yet known whether similar neurobiological alterations underlie simple MND. But the finding that simple MND is associated with a slightly increased prevalence of learning and behavioural problems, in particular attention problems and externalizing behaviour (Hadders-Algra, 2002; Batstra et al, 2003), suggests that altered settings in the monoaminergic systems may contribute to simple MND.

Complex MND
The data from the Groningen Perinatal Project and more recent data indicate that 6–7% of school-age children show complex MND (Hadders-Algra, 2002; Peters et al, 2010).

This means that the prevalence of complex MND, unlike that of simple MND, has not changed during the last few decades. Complex MND is clearly associated with prenatal, perinatal, and neonatal adversities and with neonatal neurological deviancy and serious lesions of the brain detected in the neonatal period (Hadders-Algra, 2002; Barnett et al, 2002; Arnaud et al, 2007). The resemblance of the aetiology of complex MND to that of cerebral palsy suggests that complex MND, from an aetiological point of view, may be regarded as a borderline form of cerebral palsy. Both cerebral palsy and complex MND are often the result of a chain of prenatal and perinatal adversities (Stanley et al, 2000; Hadders-Algra, 2002), a finding that is in line with the older concept of Knobloch and Pasamanick (1959) of 'the continuum of reproductive casualty'. Also major events occurring in isolation, such as neonatal stroke, may give rise to cerebral palsy and complex MND (Barnett et al, 2002). It should be realized, however, that not all prenatal adversities are noticed clinically. As a result a small proportion of children born at term after a seemingly uneventful pregnancy and an uncomplicated birth develop cerebral palsy or complex MND. On the basis of the aetiological analogy with cerebral palsy it may be hypothesized that complex MND is an umbrella term describing a group of children with subtle deviations in the brain that occurred during the prenatal, perinatal, or neonatal period (cf. Rosenbaum et al, 2007). Most likely the timing of the occurrence and the site of the small lesions in the children with complex MND is equally diverse as that in children with cerebral palsy. Studies applying neuroimaging techniques with a high resolution are required to test these hypotheses.

Complex MND is more strongly associated with learning, behavioural, and motor problems than simple MND (Hadders-Algra, 2002). In particular learning problems, such as difficulties in reading, spelling, and arithmetic; motor problems (indicated by a performance on the Movement ABC below the fifth centile); dysgraphic writing; attention problems and autism-spectrum disorder (ASD) are related to the presence of complex MND (Hadders-Algra, 2002; Batstra et al, 2003; Punt et al, 2010; Van Hoorn et al, 2010; Peters et al, 2010; De Jong et al, personal communication). Internalizing behaviour shows a weak association with complex MND, whereas externalizing behaviour is not associated with complex MND but rather with simple MND (Batstra et al, 2003). The latter corresponds to the finding of Breslau et al (2000) that internalizing behaviour in low-birthweight infants is more closely related to the presence of soft signs than externalizing behaviour. The notion that learning difficulties are more closely related to complex MND than behavioural problems is in line with Rutter's conclusion (1982) that mild or subclinical forms of damage to the developing brain are associated in particular with an increased risk for cognitive dysfunction and less clearly with an increased risk for behavioural disorders.

The distinction between the two forms of MND is clinically useful. The two forms have a different aetiology and they indicate a different vulnerability to learning, behavioural, and motor problems. Whether or not a child with a specific neurological condition will develop learning, behavioural, or motor problems depends on many contextual factors, including socioecomonic status, housing conditions, the presence of family adversity, the educational skills of caregivers, the presence of siblings, and that of peers.

Specific types of MND

Dysfunctional posture and muscle tone regulation
Mild dysfunctions in muscle tone regulation which are associated with mild deviations in the child's posture are regarded as a form of MND. The most commonly observed mild dysfunction is a mild diffuse hypotonia that is associated with a collapsed posture during sitting, difficulties in maintaining arm position during the posture with extended arms in supination, and an increased lumbar lordosis during standing and – less often – during walking. In children born preterm the finding of a mildly varying muscle tone is not uncommon (see Chapter 4). Mild hypertonia is a relatively rare form of MND. Mild dysfunctions in posture and muscle tone regulation occur in about 10% of children (Batstra et al, 2003, Peters et al, 2010).

The aspect of posture evaluated in this domain relies more on the static than the dynamic aspects of postural control. The dynamic aspects of postural control are assessed in particular in the domain of coordination. Both static and dynamic aspects of postural control involve virtually all parts of the nervous system (Latash and Hadders-Algra, 2008).

The clinical finding that abnormalities in muscle tone regulation may be found in disorders affecting the spinal cord, brainstem, cerebellum, basal ganglia, and the cerebral cortex (Swaiman and Ashwal, 1999) indicates that mild abnormalities in muscle tone regulation may be regarded as a relatively unspecific expression of neurological dysfunction. This is reflected by the finding that dysfunctional posture and muscle tone regulation is not related to behavioural problems and dysgraphic writing, and less clearly associated with learning difficulties and a poor performance on the Movement ABC than dysfunctions in the domains of coordination and fine manipulative ability (Batstra et al, 2003; Van Hoorn et al, 2010; Peters et al, 2010).

Mild dyskinesia
The most frequently occurring mild dyskinesia is choreiform dyskinesia. The prevalence of choreiform movements depends on the child's age. Choreiform movements are not observed in 2- to 3-year-olds. From about 4 years their prevalence increases until the age of 8. After the age of 8 years the prevalence decreases (Prechtl, 1987). Currently marked choreiform dyskinesia is observed less often than in the 1950s and 1960s (see Chapter 5). The decrease in prevalence may be related to improved perinatal care, as neonatal acidosis is one of the few obstetric factors with a weak association with choreiform dyskinesia (Soorani-Lunging et al, 1993).

Some athetotiform movements may be present in children below the age of 6 years. In older children athetotiform movements and tremors are rarely observed forms of MND.

It is tempting to speculate that choreiform and athetotiform dyskinesia are based on mild dysfunction of the basal ganglia as their serious counterparts chorea and athetosis are attributed to failure or dysfunction of these structures (Sanger and Mink, 2006). However, data to support this structural–functional relationship are missing.

Nevertheless, the finding that choreiform dyskinesia is clearly associated with attention problems, weakly with externalizing behaviour, and not at all with internalizing behaviour (Batstra et al, 2003) fits with a striatal origin to this form of dyskinesia.

Mild problems in coordination
The prevalence of mild coordination problems has increased over the last few decades. In particular the prevalence of children who are not able to perform diadochokinesis in an age-appropriate way has risen steeply (personal observation). As a result of this we decided to change the criterion for dysfunction in the domain of coordination problems from two tests inappropriate for age to three tests inappropriate for age (Peters et al, 2008). Nevertheless, the prevalence of coordination problems rose from about 4% in school-age children born in the 1970s (old criterion; De Jong et al, personal communication; Punt et al, 2010) to 15% of current school-age children (new criterion; Peters et al, 2010).

Coordination problems are associated with dysfunction of the cerebellum (Swaiman and Ashwalk, 1999; Manto, 2008). Interestingly, the cerebellum is the part of the brain with a specific developmental growth curve: its growth spurt starts later (third trimester) than that of the cerebral cortex (first half of gestation) and its growth spurt ends relatively early, i.e. around the end of the first postnatal year (Dobbing, 1974; Volpe, 2009; see also Figure 1.1). This means that the cerebellum has a different window of vulnerability than the cerebral cortex. Whether or not the significant increase in coordination problems during the last few decades is related to this specific window of cerebellar vulnerability is unknown. But it is known that very preterm birth is associated with coordination problems and cerebellar abnormalities (Soorani-Lunsing et al, 1993; Volpe, 2009).

Originally the cerebellum was only associated with motor dyscoordination, but more recently it became clear that the cerebellum may also be involved in cognitive disorders and neuropsychiatric disorders including attention deficits (Adams et al, 1974; Nichols and Chen, 1981; Steinlin, 2007; Haarmeier and Their, 2007; Hoppenbrouwers et al, 2008). Indeed, dysfunction in the domain of coordination has not only been associated with a poor performance on the Movement ABC and dysgraphia, but also with learning disorders, ASD, attention problems, and externalizing behaviour (Batstra et al, 2003; Punt et al, 2010; Van Hoorn et al, 2010; De Jong et al, personal communication; Peters et al, 2010).

Mild problems in fine manipulative ability
The domain of fine manipulative disability is based on the child's performance on three tests: the finger opposition test, the follow-a-finger test and the circle test. The presence of the follow-a-finger test and the circle test in the domain of fine manipulative ability may seem counterintuitive, as the movements involved are not small and fine. Yet, the three tests are clustered into one domain as performance on these tests largely depends on widespread activity in the cerebral cortex, including the communication between both cerebral hemispheres (Gordon et al, 1998; Eliassen et al, 1999; Kennerley et al, 2002; Wu and Hallett, 2005).

The prevalence of fine manipulative disability has remained stable over the years. It occurs in about 7% of school-age children (Punt et al, 2010; Peters et al, 2010). Considering the notion that the domain of fine manipulative ability reflects function of widespread activity in the cerebral cortex it is not so surprising that fine manipulative disability is not only strongly associated with motor problems but also with learning disorders (Batstra et al, 2003; Van Hoorn et al, 2010; Peters et al, 2010). In addition associations have been reported between fine manipulative disability and ASD, attention problems, and to a lesser extent, internalizing behaviour (Vitiello et al,1990; Batstra et al, 2003; Punt et al, 2010; De Jong et al, personal communication).

Excessive associated movements
Associated movements are movements accompanying voluntary movements. They should be distinguished from mirror movements. 'Associated movements' refers to involuntary movements in non-homologous muscles, for instance in contralateral limbs (mirror-like activity) or in other parts of the body, whereas 'mirror movements' refers to involuntary movements in homologous muscles contralateral to the involuntary movements (Hoy et al, 2004). Associated movements are part and parcel of typical development whereas mirror movements reflect atypical development (Reitz and Müller, 1998; Kuthz-Buschbeck et al, 2000). The neurophysiological mechanisms underlying associated movements are poorly understood (Hoy et al, 2004). Most likely the associated movements are produced by simultaneous activation of crossed corticospinal pathways originating from both left and right motor cortices (Mayston et al, 1999).

Associated movement activity is characterized by variation: variation between children and variation within children (Wolff et al, 1983; Vitiello et al, 1989; Gasser et al, 2007, 2009). Children may show excessive associated activity during one task but none during another. Nevertheless it is also clear that associated movements become less prominent with increasing age (Connolly and Stratton, 1968; Lazarus and Todor, 1987; Gasser et al, 2007, 2009). This may be related to an increasing influence of transcallosal inhibitory activity (Mayston et al, 1999).

The degree to which associated movements may be observed is not only related to the child's age, but also to the nature of the task. More complex tasks and tasks requiring more effort and more force are associated with more associated activity (Connolly and Stratton, 1968; Szatmari and Taylor, 1984; Lazarus and Todor, 1987; Gasser et al, 2009). Interestingly, girls show less associated activity than boys (Connolly and Stratton, 1968; Gasser et al, 2007, 2009). It is not clear whether the difference between the sexes is attributed to the complex and subtle differences in brain development between boys and girls (Durston et al, 2001) or to the higher prevalence of MND in boys (Hadders-Algra, 2002). Neurological dysfunction is known to be associated with an increased prevalence of associated activity (Abercrombie et al, 1964; Cohen et al, 1967). This association may be a direct one implying that associated activity that is excessive for age may be because of a low threshold for associated movements irrespective of task complexity. The association may also be an indirect one, i.e. it may be brought about by the fact that a child with minor dysfunction in the form of coordination problems or fine manipulative disability needs more effort to perform a task.

As a result of the large intra-individual and inter-individual variation in associated movement activity at any age the ranges for typical performance are wide. As a result the prevalence of the dysfunctional domain of excessive associated movements is low. It occurs in about 1% of children (Punt et al, 2010; Peters et al, 2010). Excessive associated movements has been reported to occur more often in children with behavioural problems (Szatmari and Taylor, 1984), ASD (De Jong et al, personal communication) and dyslexia (Punt et al, 2010).

Mild cranial nerve dysfunction
Mild cranial nerve dysfunction is a rare form of MND. The most frequently found mild palsies are a mild dysfunction of the abducens nerve or facial nerve (Hadders-Algra et al, 1986). These dysfunctions may be present as an isolated dysfunction, but most often they are found in children with many signs of MND. Mild cranial nerve dysfunction as a single phenomenon has little clinical significance, its presence appears to function mainly as a marker for the severity of MND.

Mild sensory dysfunction
Few children in mainstream education fulfil the criteria for mild sensory dysfunction. It should be realized that the tests to evaluate sensory function included in the assessment of MND are relatively insensitive. This may explain the absence of associations between the domain of sensory dysfunction and poor performance on the Movement ABC or dysgraphic handwriting tests (Van Hoorn et al, 2010; Peters et al, 2010). It is known that children with developmental coordination disorder (DCD), when measured with sensitive methods, may show signs of impaired sensory function, such as impaired proprioception (as indicated by impaired aiming movements in the absence of visual control; Smyth and Mason, 1998), impaired visual acuity (Evensen et al, 2009), impaired complex visuospatial abilities (Wilson and McKenzie 1998), and poor kinaestetic perception (Wilson and McKenzie 1998). The absence of an association between the domain of sensory dysfunction and motor impairment contrasts with the association between sensory dysfunction and ASD. A recent study indicated that about 15% of children with ASD show this dysfunction (De Jong et al, personal communication).

Application of the assessment in research
The assessment of MND is primarily a tool for clinical practice. The assessment may, however, also be applied in research. Examples of studies that have used MND as an outcome parameter include ones evaluating the association between neurological conditions and preterm birth (Hadders-Algra et al, 1988b; Fallang et al, 2005; Arnaud et al, 2007), intrauterine growth retardation (Ley et al, 1996), perinatal asphyxia (Barnett et al, 2002), neonatal neurological dysfunction (Hadders-Algra et al 1986, 1988c, Soorani-Lunsing et al, 1993), intracytoplasmatic sperm injection (Knoester et al, 2007), and postnatal supplementation with long-chain polyunsaturated fatty acids (De Jong et al, 2010). Outcome may be expressed in terms of severity or type of MND.

Neurological optimality score
The assessment of MND may also be expressed in terms of a neurological optimality score (NOS, cf. Touwen et al, 1980; Huisman et al, 1995). For the calculation of the NOS optimal ranges for the items on the neurological examination have been defined. The total number of items scored within the optimal range determines the NOS (range 0–64; Table 10.3). It is important to realize that there is a conceptual difference between typical performance and optimality as the range for optimal behaviour may be narrower than that for typical behaviour (Prechtl, 1980). As a result of this characteristic, the NOS is able to evaluate subtle differences in neurological outcome. For instance, application of the NOS at 18 months allows for the detection of a positive effect for prenatal long-chain polyunsaturated fatty acid status and a negative effect for trans-fatty acid status (Bouwstra et al, 2006).

Value in clinical practice
The assessment of MND provides information about a child's neurological condition. The neurological condition in terms of any MND helps in identifying the child's vulnerability to develop motor, learning, or behavioural problems. It is, however, important to bear in mind that neurological condition is only one factor – a factor at the level of body impairment – determining whether a child will develop limitations in motor, academic, or behavioural domains interfering with participation.

MND and therapeutic guidance
In clinical practice it is in particular the severity of MND that has clinical significance. The presence of simple MND suggests the presence of a typically, but non-optimally functioning brain. The non-optimal brain may, for example, consist of a nervous system in which the dopaminergic, serotonergic, or noradrenergic circuitries exhibit slightly altered function, a condition that interferes with the optimal adaptation of behaviour (Sara, 2009). The presence of a typical, but non-optimally functioning nervous system in children with a developmental disorder may imply that the child in general is able to achieve typical levels of activity and participation by means of training of skills, proper educational guidance, and minor adjustments to the tasks (Hadders-Algra, 2000b).

The presence of complex MND suggests that minor dysfunction is rather widespread in the nervous system. The aetiological analogy with cerebral palsy suggests that complex MND may originate from subtle structural changes in the brain that originate during the prenatal, perinatal, or neonatal period. It has been suggested that this type of brain dysfunction is associated with two problems: (1) a limited repertoire of behavioural strategies, and (2) difficulties adapting behaviour to the specifics of a situation (Hadders-Algra, 2000b). A consequence of a limited repertoire of strategies is that the child's potential to achieve specific skills has limitations (Hadders-Algra, 2000b, 2003). For children with a developmental disorder who exhibit complex MND this may mean that, in addition to training and proper educational assistance, use of medication may be considered (in children with behavioural disorders such as attention-deficit–hyperactivity disorder [ADHD]), or assistive technology. In children with a motor impairment the latter may consist for instance of the application of adapted writing utensils, the use of a

Table 10.3 Neurological optimality score (NOS, see De Jong et al, 2010)

Domain	Age, years	Criteria for optimality
Posture and muscle tone		
(1) Sitting, standing and walking	≥4	Ability to perform independently
(2) Posture while sitting	≥4	Typical posture of head, trunk, arms and legs
(3) Extending arms in pronation and supination while sitting	≥4	Ability to stabilize the arms in space
(4) Voluntary relaxation	≥4	Easy
(5) Muscle power in head, trunk, arms, and legs	≥4	Typical power for age
(6) Muscle tone of the head and trunk	≥4	Typical muscle tone
(7) Muscle tone of arms and legs	≥4	Typical muscle tone
(8) Range of the head, trunk, arms, and legs	≥4	Typical range
(9) Posture while standing	≥4	Typical posture of head, trunk, arms, and legs
(10) Posture while walking	≥4	Typical posture of head, trunk, arms, and legs
(11) Walking on toes and walking on heels	≥4	Able to walk on toes and on heels
Reflexes		
(12) Reflex threshold of biceps reflex, triceps reflex, knee jerk, and ankle jerk	≥4	All thresholds in typical range
(13) Reflex intensity of biceps reflex, triceps reflex, knee jerk, and ankle jerk	≥4	All intensities in typical range
(14) Footsole response	≥4	Symmetrical plantar flexion or no response
(15) Plantar grasp	≥4	Bilaterally absent
(16) Abdominal skin reflex	≥4	Symmetrically present
Involuntary movements		
(17) Presence of choreiform movements during sitting with or without extended arms	≥4	No

Table 10.3 Continued

Domain	Age, years	Criteria for optimality
(18) Presence of athetotiform movements during sitting with or without extended arms	≥4	No
(19) Presence of tremor during sitting with or without extended arms	≥4	No
(20) Test for involuntary movements (standing): distal choreiform movements	≥4	No
(21) Test for involuntary movements (standing): proximal choreiform movements	≥4	No
(22) Test for involuntary movements (standing): athetotiform movements	≥4	No
(23) Test for involuntary movements (standing): tremor	≥4	No
(24) Choreiform movements of the eyes during fixation and pursuit	≥4	No
(25) Choreiform movements of the face during fixation and pursuit	≥4	No
(26) Choreiform movements of the tongue while sticking out the tongue	≥4	No
Coordination and balance	≥4	
(27) Kicking (while sitting)	≥4	Typical performance
(28) Reaction to push while sitting	≥4	Typical performance
(29) Reaction to push while standing	≥4	Typical performance
(30) Romberg test	≥4	Typical performance
(31) Diadochokinesis	≥4	Typical performance
(32) Finger–nose test	≥4	Typical performance
(33) Fingertip–touching test	≥4	Typical performance
(34) Walking along a straight line	≥4	Typical performance
(35) Standing on one leg	4	Both legs ≥5 s
	5	Both legs ≥10 s
	6	Both legs ≥15 s
	7–9	Both legs ≥20 s
	≥10	Both legs ≥20 s, no toe flexion, no sway

Table 10.3 Continued

Domain	Age, years	Criteria for optimality
(36) Hopping on one leg	4	Both legs ≥5 hops
	5	Both legs ≥10 hops
	6	Both legs ≥15 hops
	7–9	Both legs ≥20 hops
	≥10	Both legs ≥20 hops, on the same spot, and on toes
(37) Knee–heel test	≥5	Typical performance
Fine manipulation		
(38) Finger opposition test: smoothness	4	Also optimal when not able to perform the test
	≥5	Typical performance
(39) Finger opposition test: transition	4	Also optimal when not able to perform the test
	≥5	Typical performance
(40) Follow-a-finger test	≥4	Typical performance
(41) Circle test: opposite directions	≥4	Typical performance
(42) Circle test: same direction	4	Also optimal when not able to perform the test
	≥5	Typical performance
(43) Circle test: transition	4	Also optimal when not able to perform the test
	≥5	Typical performance
Associated movements		
(44) Mouth-opening and finger-spreading phenomena	≥4	Typical performance
(45) Associated movements during diadochokinesis	≥4	Typical performance
(46) Associated movements during finger opposition test	4	Also optimal when not able to perform the test
	≥5	Typical performance
(47) Associated movements during walking on tiptoes	≥4	Typical performance
(48) Associated movements during walking on heels	≥4	Typical performance

Table 10.3 Continued

Domain	Age, years	Criteria for optimality
Sensory function		
(49) Graphaesthesia	4	Also optimal when not able to perform the test
	≥5	Appropriate performance
(50) Kinaesthesia	4	Also optimal when not able to perform the test
	≥5	Typical performance
(51) Sense of position	4	Also optimal when not able to perform the test
	≥5	Appropriate performance
(52) Vision	≥4	Typical, no need for visual correction
(53) Hearing	≥4	Typical performance
Cranial nerve function		
(54) Facial motility	≥4	Typical
(55) Position of the eyes	≥4	Typical
(56) Fixation of the eyes	≥4	Typical
(57) Pupillary reactions	≥4	Typical
(58) Pursuit movements of the eyes	≥4	Typical in all directions
(59) Nystagmus	≥4	Absent
(60) Visual fields	≥4	Typical
(61) Tongue motility	≥4	Typical
(62) Speech	≥4	Typical
(63) Pharyngeal arches	≥4	Typical
(64) Quality of walking	≥4	Typical

laptop for writing, or the use of adaptive seating (Hadders-Algra and Brogren Carlberg 2008; Van Hoorn et al, 2010).

The domains of dysfunction with the largest clinical importance are fine manipulative disability and coordination problems. Both of these domains reflect dysfunction of complex supraspinal circuitries. Therefore it is not very surprising that in particular these domains are most strongly associated with motor, learning, and psychiatric disorders. Mild dysfunctions in the domain of posture and muscle tone regulation only show a weak relation with developmental disorders including motor impairments. This supports the idea that therapeutic guidance for children with DCD should focus on practising complex functions used in daily life – as currently is advocated in training programmes such as cognitive orientation to daily occupational performance (CO-OP; Sangster et al, 2005) and neuromotor task training (Niemeijer et al, 2007) – rather than on muscle tone regulation as applied in neurodevelopmental treatment (Howle, 2002).

MND and prognosis
As a result of the impressive developmental changes that occur in the brain the child's neurological condition may alter over the years. A child's neurological condition may improve, it may deteriorate, or it may remain stable (Hertzig, 1982; Hadders-Algra, 2002; Schothorst et al, 2007). Nevertheless, the child who exhibits complex MND at school age has a substantially increased risk of continuing to show complex MND in adolescence (Soorani-Lunsing et al, 1993; Hadders-Algra, 2002).

Only a few studies have addressed the long-term prognosis for MND at school age. Shaffer et al (1985) reported that the severity of MND at 7 years was associated with the risk for cognitive impairment at 17 years. The study also indicated that the presence (not the severity) of minor dysfunction at 7 was related to the presence of psychiatric morbidity at 17. The association was brought about by the increased prevalence of anxious and withdrawn behaviour in children with MND at 7. The rates of conduct disorder and ADHD at age 17 were not increased in the children with MND at 7 years. Also, a study by Schothorst and colleagues (2007) indicated that the presence of MND at school age increased the risk for psychiatric morbidity at 15 to 17 years. The risk for psychiatric disorders increased especially when the signs of MND had persisted into adolescence. A study by Rasmussen and Gillberg (2000) that reported outcome at 22 years of children followed from school age with various neurodevelopmental conditions suggested that in particular children who exhibited deficits in attention, motor control and perception (DAMP), had a poor outcome in terms of school achievement, psychiatry morbidity, and criminal offence. This condition is characterized by the presence of multiple dysfunctions of the brain and children with DAMP often show complex MND (Jucaite et al, 2003). The latter findings support the suggestion that the severity of neurological dysfunction has prognostic value (Rutter, 1982).

Concluding remarks
The assessment of MND facilitates the development of an optimal therapeutic approach for children with motor, learning, and behavioural disorders. In particular the distinction into the simple and complex form of MND is clinically relevant. It is the complex form that is clearly associated with concurrent motor, learning, and behavioural problems and with an increased risk for psychiatric morbidity and school failure later in life.

References

Abercrombie MLJ, Lindon RL, Tyson MC. (1964) Associated movements in normal and physically handicapped children. *Dev Med Child Neurol* 6: 573–80.

Adams RM, Kocsis JJ, Estes RE. (1974) Soft neurological signs in learning disabled children and controls. *Am J Dis Child* 128: 614–8.

Allen MC. (2008) Neurodevelopmental outcomes of preterm infants. *Curr Opin Neurol* 21: 123–8.

American Psychiatric Association. (1980) *Diagnostic and Statistical Manual of Mental Disorder (3rd edn) (DSM–IIII)*. Washington, DC: APA.

American Psychiatric Association. (2000) *Diagnostic and Statistical Manual of Mental Disorder (4th edn) (DSM–IV)*. Washington DC: APA.

Angold A, Costello FJ, Erkanli A. (1999) Comorbidity. *J Child Psychol Psychiatry* 40: 57–87.

Annett M. (1979) Family handedness in three generations predicted by the right shift theory. *Ann Hum Genet* 42: 479–91.

Arnaud C, Daubisse-Marliac L, White-Koning M, Pierrat V, Larroque B, Grandjean H, Alberge C, Marret S, Burguet A, Ancel PY, Supernant K, Kaminski M. (2007) Prevalence and associated factors of minor neuromotor dysfunctions at age 5 years in prematurely born children: the EPIPAGE Study. *Arch Pediatr Adolesc Med* 161: 1053–61.

Babinski JF. (1902) Sur le role du cervelet dans les actes volitionnels necessitant une succession rapide de mouvements (diadococinese). *Rev Neurol* 10: 1013–5.

Baraldi P, Porro CA, Serafini M, Pagnoni G, Marari C, Corazza R, Nichelli P. (1999) Bilateral representation of sequential finger movements in human cortical areas. *Neurosci Lett* 269: 95–8.

Barlow CF. (1974) "Soft signs" in children with learning disorders. *Am J Dis Child* 128: 605–6.

Barnea-Goraly N, Menon V, Eckert M, Tamm L, Bammer R, Karchemskiy A, Dant CC, Reiss AL. (2005) White matter development during childhood and adolescence: a cross-sectional diffusion tensor imaging study. *Cereb Cortex* 15: 1848–54.

Barnett A, Mercuri E, Rutherford M, Haataja L, Frisone MF, Henderson S, Cowan F, Dubowitz L. (2002) Neurological and perceptual-motor outcome at 5–6 years of age in children with neonatal encephalopathy: relationship with neonatal brain MRI. *Neuropediatrics* 33: 242–8.

Bastian AJ. (2006) Learning to predict the future: the cerebellum adapts feedforward movement control. *Curr Opin Neurobiol* 16: 645–9.

References

Batstra L, Neeleman J, Hadders-Algra M. (2003) The neurology of learning and behavioral problems in pre-adolescent children. *Acta Psychiatr Scand* 108: 92–100.

Batstra L, Neeleman J, Elsinga C, Hadders-Algra M. (2006) Psychiatric multimorbidity in young adults is related to a chain of pre- and perinatal adversities. *Early Hum Dev* 82: 721–9.

Bax MCO, Mac Keith RC. (1963) *Minimal Cerebral Dysfunction. Clin Dev Med 10.* London: Heinemann Medical Books.

Berninger VW, Colwell SO. (1985) Relationships between neurodevelopmental and educational findings in children aged 6 to 12 years. *Pediatrics* 75: 697–702.

Boecker H, Jankowski J, Ditter P, Scheef L. (2008) A role of the basal ganglia and midbrain nuclei for initiation of motor sequences. *Neuroimage* 39: 1356–69.

Bouwstra H, Dijck-Brouwer DAJ, Decsi T, Boehm G, Boersma ER, Muskiet FAJ, Hadders-Algra M. (2006) Neurological condition at 18 months: positive association with venous umbilical DHA-status and negative association with umbilical trans-fatty acids. *Pediatr Res* 60: 1–7.

Breslau N, Chilcoat HD, Johnson EO, Andreski P, Lucia VC. (2000) Neurologic soft signs and low birthweight: their association and neuropsychiatric implications. *Biol Psychiatry* 47: 71–9.

Brown G, Chadwick O, Shaffer D, Rutter M, Traub M. (1981) A prospective study of children with head injuries: III Psychiatric sequelae. *Psychol Med* 11: 63–78.

Bruininks RH. (1978) *Bruininks-Oseretsky Test of Motor Proficiency.* Circle Pines, MN: American Guidance Service.

Cannon M, Byrne M, Cassidy B, Larkin C, Horgan R, Sheppard NP, O'Callaghan E. (1995). Prevalence and correlates of mixed-handedness in schizophrenia. *Psychiatry Res* 59: 119–25.

Capute AJ, Shapiro BK, Palmer FB. (1981) Spectrum of developmental disabilities. *Orthop Clin North Am* 12: 3–22.

Carson RG, Thomas J, Summers JJ, Walters MR, Semjen A. (1997) The dynamics of bimanual circle drawing. *Q J Exp Psychol A* 50: 664–83.

Chadwick O, Rutter M, Brown G, Shaffer D, Traub M. (1981) A prospective study of children with head injuries: II Cognitive sequelae. *Psychol Med* 11: 49–61.

Cioni G, Duchini F, Milianti B, Paolicelli PB, Sicola E, Boldrini A, Ferrari A. (1993) Differences and variations in the patterns of early independent walking. *Early Hum Dev* 35: 193–205.

Close J. (1973) Scored neurological examination in pharmacotherapy of children. *Psychopharmacol Bull* special issue (pharmacotherapy of children): 142–8.

Cohen HJ, Taft LT, Mahadeviah MS, Birch HG. (1967) Developmental changes in overflow in normal and aberrantly functioning children. *J Pediatr* 71: 39–47.

Connolly K, Stratton P. (1968) Developmental changes in associated movements. *Dev Med Child Neurol* 10: 49–56.

Contreras-Vidal JL, Bo J, Boudreau JP, Clark JE. (2005) Development of visuomotor representations for hand movement in young children. *Exp Brain Res* 162: 155–64.

Corbetta D, Thelen E. (1996) Lateral biases and fluctuations in infants' spontaneous arm movements and reaching. *Dev Psychobiol* 34: 237–55.

De Graaf-Peters VB, Hadders-Algra M. (2006) Ontogeny of the human central nervous system: what is happening when? *Early Hum Dev* 82: 257–66.

De Guise E, Lassonde M. (2001) Callosal contribution to procedural learning in children. *Dev Neuropsychol* 19: 253–72.

De Jong M, Punt M, De Groot E, Hielkema T, Struik M, Minderaa RB, Hadders-Algra M. (2009) Symptom diagnostics based on clinical records: a tool for scientific research in child psychiatry? *Eur Child Adoles Psychiatry* 18: 257–64.

De Jong C, Kikkert HK, Fidler V, Hadders-Algra M. (2010) The Groningen LCPUFA-study: effect of postnatal long-chain polyunsaturated fatty acids in healthy term infants on neurological condition at 9 years. *Br J Nutr* April 7: 1–7 (Epub ahead of print) doi:10.1017/S0007114510000863.

Denckla MB. (1973) Development of speed in repetitive and successive finger-movements in normal children. *Dev Med Child Neurol* 15: 635–45.

Denckla MB. (1974) Development of motor co-ordination in normal children. *Dev Med Child Neurol* 16: 729–41.

Denckla MB. (1985) Revised Neurological Examination for Subtle Signs (1985). *Psychopharmacol Bull* 21: 773–800.

Denckla MB, Rudel RG. (1978) Anomalies of motor development in hyperactive boys. *Ann Neurol* 3: 231–3.

De Vries AM, De Groot L. (2002) Transient dystonias revisited: a comparative study of preterm and term children at 2 1/2 years of age. *Dev Med Child Neurol* 44: 415–21.

Dietz V. (1992) Human neuronal control of automatic functional movements. Interaction between central programs and afferent input. *Physiol Rev* 72: 33–69.

Dobbing J. (1974) The later growth of the brain and its vulnerability. *Pediatrics* 53: 2–6.

Drillien CM. (1972) Abnormal neurologic signs in the first year of life in low-birthweight infants: possible prognostic significance. *Dev Med Child Neurol* 14: 575–84.

Durston S, Hulshoff Pol HE, Casey BJ, Giedd JN, Buitelaar JK, van Engeland H. (2001) Anatomical MRI of the developing human brain: what have we learned? *J Am Acad Child Adolesc Psychiatry* 40: 1012–20.

Elia J, Ambrosini P, Berrettini W. (2008) ADHD characteristics: I. Concurrent co-morbidity patterns in children & adolescents. *Child Adolesc Psychiatry Ment Health* 3: 15.

Eliassen JC, Baynes K, Gazzaniga MS. (1999) Direction information coordinated via the posterior third of the corpus callosum during bimanual movements. *Exp Brain Res* 128: 573–7.

Escolar DM, Leshner RT. (2006) Muscular dystrophies. In: Swaiman KF, Ashwal S, Ferriero DM, editors. *Pediatric Neurology, Principles and Practice (4th edn)*. Philadelphia, PA: Mosby. pp 1969–2013.

Evensen KAI, Lindqvist S, Indredavik MS, Skranes J, Brubakk AM, Vik T. (2009) Do visual impairments affect risk of motor problems in preterm and term low birth weight adolescents. *Eur J Paddiatr Neurol* 13: 47–56.

Fallang B, Saugstad OD, Hadders-Algra M. (2000) Goal directed reaching and postural control in supine position in healthy infants. *Behav Brain Res* 115: 9–18.

Fallang B, Øien I, Hellem E, Saugstad OD, Hadders-Algra M. (2005) Quality of reaching and postural control in young preterm infants is related to neuromotor outcome at 6 years. *Pediatr Res* 58: 347–53.

Farmer SE. (2003) Key factors in the development of lower limb co-ordination: implications for the acquisition of walking in children with cerebral palsy. *Disabil Rehabil* 25: 807–16.

Fellick JM, Thomson APJ, Sills J, Hart CA. (2001) Neurological soft signs in mainstream pupils. *Arch Dis Child* 85: 371–4.

Flitcroft DI, Adams GG, Robson AG, Holder GE. (2005) Retinal dysfunction and refractive errors: an electrophysiological study of children. *Br J Ophthalmol* 89: 484–8.

Fleuren KM, Smit LS, Stijnen T, Hartman A. (2007). New reference values for the Alberta Infant Motor Scale need to be established. *Acta Paediatr* 96: 424–7.

Freitag CM, Kleser C, Schneider M, von Gontard A. (2007) Quantitative assessment of neuromotor function in adolescents with high functioning autism and Asperger Syndrome. *J Autism Dev Disord* 37: 948–59.

Fryer SK, Frank LR, Spadoni AD, Theilmann RJ, Nagel BJ, Schweinsburg AD, Tapert SF. (2008) Microstructural integrity of the corpus callosum linked with neuropsychological performance in adolescents. *Brain Cogn* 67: 225–33.

Gardner-Medwin D, Johnston HM. (1984) Severe muscular dystrophy in girls. *J Neurol Sci* 64: 79–87.

Gasser T, Rousson V, Caflisch J, Jenni OG. (2009) Development of motor speed and associated movements from 5 to 18 years. *Dev Med Child Neurol* 52: 256–63.

Gasser T, Rousson V, Caflisch J, Largo R. (2007) Quantitative reference curves for associated movements in children and adolescents. *Dev Med Child Neurol* 49: 608–14.

Gesell A, Ames LB. (1947) The development of handedness. *J Genet Psychol* 70: 155–75.

References

Gillberg C, Kadesjö B. (2003) Why bother about clumsiness? The implications of having developmental coordination disorder (DCD). *Neural Plast* 10: 59–68.

Goez H, Zelnik N. (2008) Handedness in patients with developmental coordination disorder. *J Child Neurol* 23: 151–4.

Goodale MA, Westwood DA. (2004) An evolving view of duplex vision: separate but interacting cortical pathways for perception and action. *Curr Opin Neurobiol* 14: 203–11.

Gordon AM, Lee JH, Flament D, Ugurbil K, Ebner TJ. (1998) Functional magnetic resonance imaging of motor, sensory, and posterior parietal cortical areas during performance of sequential typing movements. *Exp Brain Res* 121: 153–66.

Groen SE, de Blécourt ACE, Postema K, Hadders-Algra M. (2005) Quality of general movements predicts neuromotor development at the age of 9–12 years. *Dev Med Child Neurol* 47: 731–8.

Haarmeier T, Thier P. (2007) The attentive cerebellum—myth or reality. *Cerebellum* 6: 177–83.

Hadders-Algra M. (2000a) The Neuronal Group Selection Theory: an attractive framework to explain variation in normal motor development. *Dev Med Child Neurol* 42: 566–72.

Hadders-Algra M. (2000b) The Neuronal Group Selection Theory: promising principles for understanding and treating developmental motor disorders. *Dev Med Child Neurol* 42: 707–15.

Hadders-Algra M. (2002) Two distinct forms of minor neurological dysfunction: perspectives emerging from a review of data of the Groningen Perinatal Project. *Dev Med Child Neurol* 44: 561–71.

Hadders-Algra M. (2003) Developmental coordination disorder: is clumsy motor behaviour caused by a lesion of the brain at early age? *Neural Plast* 10: 39–50.

Hadders-Algra M. (2004) General movements: a window for early identification of children at high risk of developmental disorders. *J Pediatr* 145: S12–8.

Hadders-Algra M. (2007) Atypical performance: how do we deal with that? *Dev Med Child Neurol* 49: 323.

Hadders-Algra M, Brogren Carlberg E. (2008) *Postural Control: A Key Issue in Developmental Disorders. Clin Dev Med 179*. London: Mac Keith Press.

Hadders-Algra M, Touwen BCL, Huisjes HJ. (1986) Neurologically deviant newborns: neurological and behavioural development at the age of six years. *Dev Med Child Neurol* 28: 569–78.

Hadders-Algra M, Huisjes HJ, Touwen BCL. (1988a) Perinatal risk factors and minor neurological dysfunction: significance for behaviour and school achievement at nine years. *Dev Med Child Neurol* 30: 482–91.

Hadders-Algra M, Huisjes HJ, Touwen BCL. (1988b) Preterm or small-for-gestational-age infants. Neurological and behavioural development at the age of 6 years. *Eur J Pediatr* 147: 460–7.

Hadders-Algra M, Huisjes HJ, Touwen BCL. (1988c) Perinatal correlates of major and minor neurological dysfunction at schoolage – a multivariate analysis. *Dev Med Child Neurol* 30: 472–81.

Hadders-Algra M, Nakae Y, Van Eykern LA, Klip-Van den Nieuwendijk AWJ, Prechtl HFR. (1993) The effect of behavioural state on general movements in healthy full-term newborns. A polymyographic study. *Early Hum Dev* 35: 63–79.

Hadders-Algra M, Brogren E, Forssberg H. (1998) Development of postural control – differences between ventral and dorsal muscles? *Neurosci Biobehav Rev* 22: 501–6.

Heineman KR, Hadders-Algra M. (2008) Evaluation of neuromotor function in infancy – a systematic review of available methods. *J Dev Behav Pediatr* 29: 315–23.

Hempel MS. (1993a) Neurological development during toddling age in normal children and children at risk of developmental disorders. *Early Hum Dev* 34: 47–57.

Hempel MS. (1993b) *The Neurological Examination for Toddler-Age*. PhD-Thesis, University of Groningen.

Henderson SE, Sugden DA. (2007). *The Movement Assessment Battery for Children (2nd edn)*. London: Harcourt Assessment.

Hermsdörfer J, Goldenberg G. (2002) Ipsilesional deficits during fast diadochokinetic hand movements following unilateral brain damage. *Neuropsychologia* 40: 2100–15.

Hertzig ME. (1981) Neurological 'soft' signs in low-birthweight children. *Dev Med Child Neurol* 23: 778–91.

Hertzig ME. (1982) Stability and change in nonfocal neurologic signs. *J Am Acad Child Psychiatry* 21: 231–6.

Hertzig ME. (1987) Nonfocal neurological signs in low birthwieght children. In: Tupper DE, editor. *Soft Neurological Signs.* New York: Grune & Stratton. pp 255–78.

Hirsch G, Wagner B. (2004) The natural history of idiopathic toe-walking: a long-term follow-up of fourteen conservatively treated children. *Acta Paediatr* 93: 196–9.

Holder EW, Tarnowski KJ, Prinz RJ. (1982) Reliability of neurological soft signs in children: reevaluation of the PANESS. *J Abn Child Psychol* 10: 163–72.

Hoppenbrouwers SS, Schutter DJ, Fitzgerald PB, Chen R, Daskalakis ZJ. (2008) The role of the cerebellum in the pathophysiology and treatment of neuropsychiatric disorders: a review. *Brain Res Rev* 59: 185–200.

Howle JM. (2002) *Neuro-Developmental Treatment Approach: Theoretical Foundations and Principles of Clinical Practice.* Laguna Beach, CA: Neuro-Developmental Treatment Association.

Hoy KE, Fitzgerald PB, Bradshaw JL, Armatas CA, Georgiou-Karistianis N. (2004) Investigating the cortical origins of motor overflow. *Brain Res Brain Res Rev* 46: 315–27.

Huisman M, Koopman-Esseboom C, Lanting CI, van der Paauw CG, Tuinstra LG, Fidler V, Weisglas-Kuperus N, Sauer PJ, Boersma ER, Touwen BC. (1995) Neurological condition in 18-month-old children perinatally exposed to polychlorinated biphenyls and dioxins. *Early Hum Dev* 43: 165–76.

Ingram TTS. (1973) Soft signs. *Dev Med Child Neurol* 15: 527–30.

Jansiewicz EM, Goldberg MC, Newschaffer CJ, Denckla MB, Landa R, Mostofsky SH. (2006) Motor signs distinguish children with high functioning autism and Asperger's syndrome from controls. *J Autism Dev Disord* 36: 613–21.

Jongmans M, Henderson S, de Vries L, Dubowitz L. (1993) Duration of periventricular densities in preterm infants and neurological outcome at 6 years of age. *Arch Dis Child* 69: 9–13.

Jucaite A, Fernell E, Forssberg H, Hadders-Algra M. (2003) Deficient coordination of associated postural adjustments during a lifting task in children with neurodevelopmental disorders. *Dev Med Child Neurol* 45: 731–42.

Kakebeeke TH, Jongmans MJ, Dubowitz LM, Schoemaker MM, Henderson SE. (1993) Some aspects of the reliability of Touwen's examination of the child with minor neurological dysfunction. *Dev Med Child Neurol* 35: 1097–105.

Kalverboer AF, Van Praag HM, Medlewicz J. (1978) *Minimal Brain Dysfunction: Fact or Fiction. Advances in Biological Psychiatry (Vol. 1).* Basel: Karger.

Karachalios T, Sofianos J, Roidis N, Sapkas G, Korres D, Nikolopoulos K. (1999) Ten-year follow-up evaluation of a school screening program for scoliosis. Is the forward-bending test an accurate diagnostic criterion for the screening of scoliosis? *Spine* 24: 2318–24.

Kavounoudias A, Roll JP, Anton JL, Nazarian B, Roth M, Roll R. (2008) Proprio-tactile integration for kinesthetic perception: an fMRI study. *Neuropsychologia* 46: 567–75.

Kawi AA, Pasamanick B. (1958) Association of factors of pregnancy with reading disorders in childhood. *J Am Med Assoc* 166: 1420–3.

Kennard MA. (1960) Value of equivocal signs in neurologic diagnosis. *Neurology* 10: 753–64.

Kennerley SW, Diedrichsen J, Hazeltine E, Semjen A, Ivry RB. (2002) Callosotomy patients exhibit temporal uncoupling during continuous bimanual movements. *Nat Neurosci* 5: 376–81.

Kessler JW. (1980) History of minimal brain dysfunctions. In: Rie HE, Rie ED, editors. *Handbook of Minimal Brain Dysfunctions. A Critical View.* New York: John Wiley & Sons. pp 18–52.

Kikkert HK, Middelburg KJ, Hadders-Algra M. Maternal anxiety is related to infant neurological condition, paternal anxiety is not. *Early Hum Dev* 86: 171–7.

Knobloch H, Pasamanick B. (1959) Syndromes of minimal cerebral damage in infancy. *JAMA* 170: 1384–7.

References

Knoester M, Vandenbroucke JP, Helmerhorst FM, van der Westerlaken LA, Walther FJ, Veen S. (2007) Matched follow-up study of 5–8 year old ICSI-singletons: comparison of their neuromotor development to IVF and naturally conceived singletons. *Hum Reprod* 22: 1638–46.

Koenderink MJ, Uylings HB. (1995) Postnatal maturation of layer V pyramidal neurons in the human prefrontal cortex. A quantitative Golgi analysis. *Brain Res* 678: 233–43.

Konczak J, Dichgans J. (1997) The development toward stereotypic arm kinematics during reaching in the first 3 years of life. *Exp Brain Res* 117: 346–54.

Krägeloh-Mann I, Horber V. (2007) The role of magnetic resonance imaging in elucidating the pathogenesis of cerebral palsy: a systematic review. *Dev Med Child Neurol* 49: 144–51.

Krain AL, Castellanos FX. (2006) Brain development and ADHD. *Clin Psychol Rev* 26: 433–44.

Kuhtz-Buschbeck JP, Stolze H, Jöhnk K, Boczek-Funcke A, Illert M. (1998) Development of prehension movements in children: a kinematic study. *Exp Brain Res* 122: 424–32.

Kuhtz-Buschbeck JP, Sundholm LK, Eliasson AC, Forssberg H. (2000) Quantitative assessment of mirror movements in children and adolescents with hemiplegic cerebral palsy. *Dev Med Child Neurol* 42: 728–36.

Lacquaniti F, Perani D, Guigon E, Bettinardi V, Carrozzo M, Grassi F, Rossetti Y, Fazio F. (1997) Visuomotor transformations for reaching to memorized targets: a PET study. *Neuroimage* 5: 129–46.

Langkamp DL, Brazy JE. (1999). Risk for later school problems in preterm children who do not cooperate for preschool developmental testing. *J Pediatr* 135: 756–60.

Largo RH, Pfister D, Molinari L, Kundu S, Lipp A, Duc G. (1989) Significance of prenatal, perinatal and postnatal factors in the development of AGA preterm infants at five to seven years. *Dev Med Child Neurol* 31: 440–56.

Largo RH, Caflisch JA, Hug F, Muggli K, Molnar AA, Molinari L, Sheehy A, Gasser T. (2001a) Neuromotor development from 5 to 18 years. Part 1: timed performance. *Dev Med Child Neurol* 43: 436–43.

Largo RH, Caflisch JA, Hug F, Muggli K, Mornar AA, Molinari L. (2001b) Neuromotor development from 5 to 18 years. Part 2: associated movements. *Dev Med Child Neurol* 43: 444–53.

Latash M, Hadders-Algra M. (2008) What is posture and how is it controlled? In: Hadders-Algra M, Brogren Carlberg E, editors. *Postural Control: A Key Issue in Developmental Disorders. Clin Dev Med 179.* London: Mac Keith Press. pp 3–21.

Lazarus J-AC, Todor JI. (1987) Age differences in the magnitude of associated movement. *Dev Med Child Neurol* 29: 726–33.

Lenroot RK, Giedd JN. (2006) Brain development in children and adolescents: insights from anatomical magnetic resonance imaging. *Neurosci Biobehav Rev* 30: 718–29.

Ley D, Laurin J, Bjerre I, Marsal K. (1996) Abnormal fetal aortic velocity waveform and minor neurological dysfunction at 7 years of age. *Ultrasound Obstet Gynecol* 8: 152–9.

Li Y, Dai Q, Jackson JC, Zhang J. (2008) Overweight is associated with decreased cognitive functioning among school-age children and adolescents. *Obesity (Silver Spring)* 16: 1809–15.

Lucas AR, Rodin EA, Simson CB. (1965) Neurological assessment of children with early school problems. *Dev Med Child Neurol* 7: 145–56.

McCartney G, Hepper P. (1999) Development of lateralized behaviour in the human fetus from 12 to 27 weeks' gestation. *Dev Med Child Neurol* 41: 83–6.

Mackie RT, McCulloch DL, Saunders KJ, Day RE, Phillips S, Dutton GN. (1998) Relation between neurological status, refractive error, and visual acuity in children: a clinical study. *Dev Med Child Neurol* 40: 31–7.

Malik SI, Painter MJ. (2004) Hypotonia and weakness. In: Kliegman RM, Greenbaum LA, Lye PS, editors. *Practical Strategies in Pediatric Diagnosis and Therapy (2nd edn).* Philadelphia, PA: Elsevier. pp 651–71.

Manto M. (2008) The cerebellum, cerebellar disorders, and cerebellar research—two centuries of discoveries. *Cerebellum* 7: 505–16.

Marlow N, Roberts BL, Cooke RW. (1989) Laterality and prematurity. *Arch Dis Child* 64: 1713–6.

Marlow N, Hennessy EM, Bracewell MA, Wolke D; EPICure Study Group. (2007) Motor and executive function at 6 years of age after extremely preterm birth. *Pediatrics* 120: 793–804.

Mayston MJ, Harrison LM, Stephens JA. (1999) A neurophysiological study of mirror movements in adults and children. *Ann Neurol* 45: 583–94.

Medical Research Council of the United Kingdom. (1978) *Aids to the Examination of the Peripheral Nervous System: Memorandum No 45*. Palo Alto, CA: Pedragon House.

Menkes JH, Sarnat HB, Moser FG. (2000) Introduction: neurologic examination of the child and infant. In: Menkes JH, Sarnat HB, editors. *Child Neurology (6th edn)*. Philadelphia, PA: Lippincott, Williams & Wilkins. pp 1–32.

Miall RC, Reckess GZ, Imamizu H. (2001) The cerebellum coordinates eye and hand tracking movements. *Nat Neurosci* 4: 638–44.

Middelburg KJ, Heineman MJ, Bos AF, Hadders-Algra M. (2008) Neuromotor, cognitive, language and behavioural outcome in children born following IVF or ICSI – a systematic review. *Hum Reprod Update* 14: 219–31.

Mink JW. (2003) The basal ganglia and involuntary movements: impaired inhibition of competing motor patterns. *Arch Neurol* 60: 1365–8.

Ming X, Brimacombe M, Wagner GC. (2007) Prevalence of motor impairment in autism spectrum disorders. *Brain Dev* 29: 565–70.

Molinari M, Filippini V, Leggio MG. (2002) Neuronal plasticity of the interrelated cerebellar and cortical networks. *Neuroscience* 111: 863–70.

Monson RM, Deitz J, Kartin D. (2003) The relationship between awake positioning and motor performance among infants who slept supine. *Pediatr Phys Ther* 15: 196–203.

Mostofsky SH, Rimrodt SL, Schafer JG, Boyce A, Goldberg MC, Pekar JJ, Denckla MB. (2006) Atypical motor and sensory cortex activation in attention-deficit/hyperactivity disorder: a functional magnetic resonance imaging study of simple sequential finger tapping. *Biol Psychiatry* 59: 48–56.

Nichols PL, Chen T-C. (1981) *Minimal Brain Dysfunction. A Prospective Study*. Hillsdale, NJ: Lawrence Erlbaum Associates.

Niemeijer AS, Smits-Engelsman BCM, Schoemaker MM. (2007) Neuromotor task training for children with developmental coordination disorder: a controlled trial. *Dev Med Child Neurol* 49: 406–11.

Njiokiktjien C. (2007) *Developmental Dyspraxias and Related Motor Disorders. Neural Substrates and Assessment*. Amsterdam: Suyi Publications.

O'Callaghan MJ, Burn YR, Mohay HA, Rogers Y, Tudehope DI. (1993) The prevalence and origins of left hand preference in high risk infants, and its implications for intellectual, motor and behavioural performance at four and six years. *Cortex* 29: 629–37.

O'Connor AR, Fielder AR. (2007) Visual outcomes and perinatal adversity. *Semin Fetal Neonatal Med* 12: 408–14.

Olsén P, Pääkkö E, Vainionpää L, Pyhtinen J, Järvelin MR. (1997) Magnetic resonance imaging of periventricular leukomalacia and its clinical correlation in children. *Ann Neurol* 41: 754–61.

Pasamanick B, Rogers ME, Lilienfeld AM. (1956) Pregnancy experience and the development of behavior disorder in children. *Am J Psychiatry* 112: 613–8.

Perelle IB, Ehrman L. (1994) An international study of human handedness: the data. *Behav Genet* 24: 217–27.

Pernet CR, Poline JB, Demonet JF, Rousselet GA. (2009) Brain classification reveals the right cerebellum as the best biomarker of dyslexia. *BMC Neurosci* 10: 67.

Peters LHJ, Maathuis KGB, Kouw E, Hamming M, Hadders-Algra M. (2008) Test-retest, inter-assessor and intra-assessor reliability of the Touwen examination. *Eur J Pediatr Neurol* 12: 328–33.

Peters LHJ, Maathuis, CGB, Hadders-Algra M. (2010) Limited motor performance and minor neurological dysfunction at school age. *Acta Paediatr* (Epub ahead of print) doi: 10.1111/j.1651-2227.2010.01998.x.

Platt MJ, Krageloh-Mann I, Cans C. (2009) Surveillance of cerebral palsy in Europe: reference and training manual. *Med Educ* 43: 495–6.

References

Prechtl HFR. (1972) Patterns of reflex behavior related to sleep in the human infant. In: Clemente C, Purpura D, Meyer F, editors. *Sleep and the Maturing Nervous System.* New York: Academic Press. pp 287–301.

Prechtl HFR. (1974) The behavioural states of the newborn infant (a review). *Brain Res* 76: 185–212.

Prechtl HFR. (1977) *The Neurological Examination of Full-Term Newborn Infant (2nd edn). Clin Dev Med 63.* London: Heinemann Medical Books.

Prechtl HFR. (1980) The optimality concept. *Early Hum Dev* 4: 201–5.

Prechtl HFR. (1987) Choreiform movements. In: Tupper DE, editor. *Soft Neurological Signs.* Orlando, FL: Grune & Stratton. pp 247–53.

Prechtl HFR. (1990) Qualitative changes of spontaneous movements in fetus and preterm infant are a marker of neurological dysfunction. *Early Hum Dev* 23: 151–8.

Prechtl HFR. (2001) General movement assessment as a method of developmental neurology: new paradigms and their consequences. *Dev Med Child Neurol* 43: 836–42.

Prechtl HFR, Stemmer C. (1962) The choreiform syndrome in children. *Dev Med Child Neurol* 4: 199–227.

Punt M, De Jong M, De Groot E, Hadders-Algra M. (2010) Minor neurological dysfunction in children with dyslexia. *Dev Med Child Neurol* (Epub ahead of print) doi: 10.1111/j.1469-8749.2010.03712.

Radovanovic S, Korotkov A, Ljubisavljevic M, Lyskov E, Thunberg J, Kataeva G, Danko S, Roudas M, Pakhomov S, Medvedev S, Johansson H. (2002) Comparison of brain activity during different types of proprioceptive inputs: a positron emission tomography study. *Exp Brain Res* 143: 276–85.

Rasmussen P, Gillberg C. (2000) Natural outcome of ADHD with developmental coordination disorder at age 22 years: a controlled, longitudinal, community-based study. *J Am Acad Child Adolesc Psychiatry* 39: 1424–31.

Reitz M, Müller K. (1998) Differences between 'congenital mirror movements' and 'associated movements' in normal children: a neurophysiological study. *Neurosci Lett* 256: 69–72.

Rie HE, Rie ED. (1980) *Handbook of Minimal Brain Dysfunctions. A Critical View.* New York: John Wiley & Sons.

Roberton MA, Halverson LE. (1988) The development of locomotor coordination: longitudinal change and invariance. *J Mot Behav* 20: 197–241.

Rochat P. (1998) Self-perception and action in infancy. *Exp Brain Res* 123: 102–9.

Rodriguez A, Waldenström U. (2008) Fetal origins of child non-right-handedness and mental health. *J Child Psychol Psychiatry* 49: 967–76.

Roncesvalles MN, Schitz C, Zedka M, Assaiante C, Woollacott M. (2005) From egocentric to exocentric spatial orientation: development of posture control in bimanual and trunk inclination tasks. *J Mot Behav* 37: 404–16.

Rosenbaum P, Paneth N, Leviton A, Goldstein M, Bax M, Damiano D, Dan B, Jacobsson B. (2007) A report: the definition and classification of cerebral palsy. *Dev Med Child Neurol* suppl 109: 8–14.

Rousson V, Gasser T, Caflisch J, Largo R. (2008) Reliability of the Zurich Neuromotor Assessment. *Clin Neuropsychol* 22: 60–72.

Rutter M. (1982) Developmental neuropsychiatry: concepts, issues and prospects. *J Clin Neuropsychol* 4: 91–115.

Rutter M, Graham P, Birch HG. (1966) Interrelations between the choreiform syndrome, reading disability and psychiatric disorders in children of 8–11 year. *Dev Med Child Neurol* 8: 149–59.

Rutter M, Graham P, Yule W. (1970) *A Neuropsychiatric Study in Childhood. Clin Dev Med 35/36.* London: Spastics International Medical Publications.

Rutter M, Chadwick O, Shaffer D, Brown G. (1980) A prospective study of children with head injuries: I Design and methods. *Psychol Med* 10: 633–45.

Sala DA, Shulman LH, Kennedy RF, Grant AD, Chu MLY. (1999) Idiopathic toe-walking: a review. *Dev Med Child Neurol* 41: 846–8.

Sanger TD, Mink JW. (2006) Movement disorders. In: Swaiman KF, Ashwal S, Ferriero DM, editors. *Pediatric Neurology, Principles and Practice (4th edn).* Philadelphia, PA: Mosby. pp 1271–311.

Sangster CA, Beninger C, Polatajko HJ, Mandich A. (2005) Cognitive strategy generation in children with developmental coordination disorder. *Can J Occup Ther* 72: 67–77.

Sara SJ. (2009) The locus coeruleus and noradrenergic modulation of cognition. *Nat Rev Neurosci* 10: 211–23.

Schaafsma SM, Riedstra BJ, Pfannkuche KA, Bouma A, Groothuis TG. (2009) Epigenesis of behavioural lateralization in humans and other animals. *Philos Trans R Soc Lond B Biol Sci* 364: 915–27.

Schmidhauser J, Caflisch J, Rousson V, Bucher HU, Largo RH, Latal B. (2006) Impaired motor performance and movement quality in very-low-birthweight children at 6 years of age. *Dev Med Child Neurol* 48:718–22.

Schmitt BD. (1975) The minimal brain dysfunction myth. *Am J Dis Child* 129: 1313–8.

Schothorst PF, Swaab-Barneveld H, van Engeland H. (2007) Psychiatric disorders and MND in non-handicapped preterm children. Prevalence and stability from school age into adolescence. *Eur Child Adolesc Psychiatry* 16: 439–48.

Shaffer D, O'Connor PA, Shafer SQ, Prupis S. (1984) Neurological 'soft signs': their origins and significance for behavior. In: Rutter M, editor. *Developmental Neuropsychiatry*. Edinburgh: Churchill Livingstone. pp 144–63.

Shaffer D, Schonfeld I, O'Connor PA, Stokman C, Trautman P, Shafer S, Ng S. (1985) Neurological soft signs. Their relationship to psychiatric disorder and intelligence in childhood and adolescence. *Arch Gen Psychiatry* 42: 342–51.

Shapiro T, Burkes L, Pett TA, Ranz J. (1978) Consistency of "nonfocal" neurological signs. *J Am Acad Child Psychiatry* 17: 70–9.

Schlotz W, Phillips DI. (2009) Fetal origins of mental health: evidence and mechanisms. *Brain Behav Immun* 23: 905–16.

Smyth MM, Mason UC. (1998) Use proprioception in normal and clumsy children. *Dev Med Child Neurol* 40: 672–81.

Sommerfelt K, Markestad T, Ellertsen B. (1998) Neuropsychological performance in low birth weight preschoolers: a population-based, controlled study. *Eur J Pediatr* 157: 53–8.

Soorani-Lunsing RJ, Hadders-Algra M, Olinga AA, Huisjes HJ, Touwen BCL. (1993) Minor neurological dysfunction after the onset of puberty: association with perinatal events. *Early Hum Dev* 33: 71–80.

Soorani-Lunsing RJ, Hadders-Algra M, Huisjes HJ, Touwen BCL. (1994) Neurobehavioural relationships after the onset of puberty. *Dev Med Child Neurol* 36: 334–43.

Sowell ER, Thompson PM, Leonard CM, Welcome SE, Kan E, Toga AW. (2004) Longitudinal mapping of cortical thickness and brain growth in normal children. *J Neurosci* 24: 8223–31.

Sprich-Buckminster S, Biederman J, Milberger S, Faraone SV, Krifcher Lehman B. (1993) Are perinatal complications relevant to the manifestation of ADD. Issue of comorbidity and familiality. *J Am Acad Child Adolesc Psychiatry* 32: 1032–7.

Stam J, Van Crevel H. (1989) Measurement of tendon reflexes by surface electromyography in normal subjects. *J Neurol* 236: 231–7.

Stanćák A, Cohen ER, Seidler RD, Duong TQ, Kim SG. (2003) The size of corpus callosum correlates with functional activation of medial motor cortical areas in bimanual and unimanual movements. *Cereb Cortex* 13: 475–85.

Stanley F, Blair E, Alberman E. (2000) *Cerebral Palsies: Epidemiology and Causal Pathways. Clin Dev Med 151.* London: Mac Keith Press.

Steinhausen HC. (2009) The heterogeneity of causes and courses of attention-deficit/hyperactivity disorder. *Acta Psychiatr Scand* 120: 392–9.

Steinlin M (2007) The cerebellum in cognitive processes: supporting studies in children. *Cerebellum* 6: 237–41.

Stephenson JBP. (2001) Commentary – soft signs: soft neurologist. *Arch Dis Child* 85: 374.

Stine OC, Saratsiotis JB, Mosser RS. (1975) Relationships between neurological findings and classroom behavior. *Am J Dis Child* 129: 1036–40.

References

Stokman CJ, Shafer SQ, Shaffer D, Ng SK, O'Connor PA, Wolff RR. (1986) Assessment of neurological 'soft signs' in adolescents: reliability studies. *Dev Med Child Neurol* 28: 428–39.

Strauss AA, Lehtinen V. (1947) *Psychopathology and Education or the Brain-Injured Child (Vol 1)*. New York: Grune & Stratton.

Sutherland DH, Olshen RA, Biden EN, Wyatt MP. (1988) *The Development of Mature Walking. Clin Dev Med 104/105*. London: Mac Keith Press.

Swaiman KE. (1999) Neurologic examination of the older child. In: Swaiman KE, Ashwal S, editors. *Pediatric Neurology. Principles and Practice (3rd edn)*. St. Louis, MO: Mosby. pp 14–30.

Swaiman KE, Ashwal S. (1999) *Pediatric Neurology. Principles and Practice (3rd edn)*. St. Louis, MO: Mosby.

Szatmari P, Taylor DC. (1984) Overflow movements and behaviour problems: scoring and using a modification of Fog's test. *Dev Med Child Neurol* 26: 297–310.

Tieman BL, Palisano RJ, Sutlive AC. (2005) Assessment of motor development and function in preschool children. *Ment Retard Dev Disabil Res Rev* 11: 189–96.

Touwen BCL. (1978) Variability and stereotypy in normal and deviant development. In: Apley J, editor. *Care of the Handicapped Child. Clin Dev Med 67*. London: Spastics International Medical Publications. pp 99–110.

Touwen BCL. (1979) *Examination of the Child with Minor Neurological Dysfunction (2nd ed). Clin Dev Med 71*. London: Spastics International Medical Publications.

Touwen BCL. (1981) Neurological development of the infant. In: Davis JA, Dobbing J, editors. *Scientific Foundations of Paediatrics (2nd edn)*. London: Heinemann Medical Books. pp 830–42.

Touwen BCL. (1993) How normal is variable, or now variable is normal? *Early Hum Dev* 34: 1–12.

Touwen BCL, Prechtl HFR. (1970) *Examination of the Child with Minor Neurological Dysfunction. Clin Dev Med 38*. London: Spastics International Medical Publications.

Touwen BCL, Sporrel T. (1979) Soft signs and MBD. *Dev Med Child Neurol* 21: 528–30.

Touwen BC, Huisjes HJ, Jurgens-van der Zee AD, Bierman-van Eendenburg ME, Smrkovsky M, Olinga AA. (1980) Obstetrical condition and neonatal neurological morbidity. An analysis with the help of the optimality concept. *Early Hum Dev* 4: 207–28.

Tracy JI, Faro SS, Mohammed FB, Pinus AB, Madi SM, Laskas JW. (2001) Cerebellar mediation of the complexity of bimanual compared to unimanual movements. *Neurology* 57: 1862–9.

Tupper DE. (1987) *Soft Neurological Signs*. New York: Grune & Stratton.

van Duijvenvoorde AC, Zanolie K, Rombouts SA, Raijmakers ME, Crone EA. (2008) Evaluating the negative or valuing the positive? Neural mechanisms supporting feedback-based learning across development. *J Neurosci* 28: 9495–503.

Van Hoorn JF, Maathuis CGB, Peters LHJ, Hadders-Algra M. (2010) Handwriting, visuomotor integration and neurological condition at school age. *Dev Med Child Neurol* (Epub ahead of print) doi: 10.1111/j.1469-8749.2010.03715.

Ververs IAP, De Vries JIP, Van Geijn HP, Hopkins B. (1994) Prenatal head position form 12–38 weeks. I. Developmental aspects. *Early Hum Dev* 39: 83–91.

Vitiello B, Ricciuti AJ, Stoff DM, Behar D, Denckla MB. (1989) Reliability of subtle (soft) neurological signs in children. *J Am Acad Child Adolesc Psychiatry* 28: 749–53.

Vitiello B, Stoff D, Atkins M, Mahoney A. (1990) Soft neurological signs and impulsivity in children. *J Dev Behav Pediatr* 11: 112–5.

Vles JSH, Van Oostenbrugge R. (1988) Head position in low-risk premature infants: impact of nursing routines. *Biol Neonate* 54: 307–13.

Volpe JJ. (2009) Cerebellum of the premature infant: rapidly developing, vulnerable, clinically important. *J Child Neurol* 24: 1085–104.

Von Hofsten C. (1991) Structuring of early reaching movements: a longitudinal study. *J Mot Behav* 23: 280–92.

Weinstock M. (2001) Alterations induced by gestational stress in brain morphology and behaviour of the offspring. *Progr Neurobiol* 65: 427–51.

Werry JS, Aman MG. (1976) The reliability and diagnostic validity of the physical and neurological examination for soft signs (PANESS). *J Autism Child Schizophr* 6: 253–62.

Wessel K, Nitschke MF. (1997) Cerebellar somatotopic representation and cerebro-cerebellar interconnections. *Prog Brain Res* 114: 577–88.

Wilke M, Krägeloh-Mann I, Holland SK. (2007) Global and local development of gray and white matter volume in normal children and adolescents. *Exp Brain Res* 178: 296–307.

Wilson PH, McKenzie BE. (1998) Information processing deficits associated with developmental coordination disorder: a meta-analysis of research findings. *J Child Psychol Psychiat* 6: 829–40.

Wocadlo C, Rieger I. (2000) Very preterm children who do not cooperate with assessments at three years of age: skill differences at 5 years. *J Dev Behav Pediatr* 21: 107–13.

Wolf DS, Singer HS. (2008) Pediatric movement disorders: an update. *Curr Opin Neurol* 21: 491–6.

Wolff PH, Hurwitz I. (1966) The choreiform syndrome. *Dev Med Child Neurol* 8: 160–5.

Wolff PH, Gunnoe CE, Cohen C. (1983) Associated movements as a measure of developmental age. *Dev Med Child Neurol* 25: 417–29.

World Health Organization. (2007) *International Classification of Functioning, Disability and Health, Child and Youth Version.* Geneva: WHO.

Wu G, Siegler S, Allard P, Kirtley C, Leardini A, Rosenbaum D, Whittle M, D'Lima D, Cristofolini L, Witte H, Schmid O, Stokes I; Standardization and Terminology Committee of the International Society of Biomechanics. (2002). ISB recommendation on definitions of joint coordinate system of various joints for the reporting of human joint motion—part I: ankle, hip, and spine. *J Biomech* 35: 543–8.

Wu G, van der Helm FC, Veeger HE, Makhsous M, Van Roy P, Anglin C, Nagels J, Karduna AR, McQuade K, Wang X, Werner FW, Buchholz B, International Society of Biomechanics. (2005) ISB recommendation on definitions of joint coordinate systems of various joints for the reporting of human joint motion—Part II: shoulder, elbow, wrist and hand. *J Biomech* 38: 981–92.

Wu T, Hallett M. (2005) The influence of normal human ageing on automatic movements. *J Physiol* 562: 605–15.

Index

Index